Contents

Preface

Over 90 years ago, Joseph H. Pilates (pronounced "puh-LAH-teez") developed a unique and revolutionary approach to physical fitness. Believing that "physical fitness is the first requisite of happiness" (Pilates and Miller 1998, p. 6), Joseph Pilates devised a series of controlled movements to engage the mind and body in developing strong, flexible muscles. Used as a method for rehabilitating injured soldiers during World War I, this new form of exercise developed a strong and faithful following among the dance community in New York City during the 1920s. Early participants marveled at how injuries healed as a result of practicing the Pilates exercises. However, it wasn't until late in the 20th century that Pilates gained widespread recognition as a viable exercise program in mainstream America.

Today, the Pilates method is enjoying a growth in popularity; it is endorsed by celebrities and athletes, and it is practiced in fitness facilities and homes across the country. Often referred to as a *mind–body* form of exercise, Pilates helps individuals become more mindful while exercising, primarily by emphasizing controlled breathing during movement and by focusing on what the body is doing. Pilates workouts leave participants feeling invigorated, serene, and self-aware—not exhausted, sore, or depleted. The exercises focus on developing strength, flexibility, and stability in the core musculature of the body—the muscles of the torso or abdomen and back—to build a foundation from which to rebalance and

realign the body. Developing these important postural muscles makes for fluid and more efficient movement, decreases risk of injury, and improves posture.

According to the U.S. Bureau of the Census (2000), there will be 70 million people over age 65 by the year 2030, more than twice the number in 1998. Many of these aging baby boomers, who are largely responsible for the fitness boom in America, intend to stay active as long as their aging bodies will let them. To extend their active years, many are exploring mind–body exercise programs such as yoga, tai chi, and Pilates. These programs also help them to reduce stress on the body, move with a more relaxed pace, and develop a more mindful focus during exercise.

The YMCA Pilates program aims to take advantage of these and many other positive aspects of Pilates exercise and bring them to local YMCAs and the communities they serve. It is a collaborative effort between YMCA of the USA and Pilates exercise experts, combining specialty exercise program expertise with the YMCA's ability to reach the community with its fitness programming. This manual contains specific information on Pilates exercise techniques, program background and philosophical information, and suggested mat exercise formats for classes.

Chapter 1 includes a discussion of Pilates as a YMCA health and fitness program and suggestions for starting a Pilates program at a local YMCA. Chapter 2 presents the history and basic concepts of Pilates exercise. Chapters 3 and 4 provide an overview of the Pilates philosophy and information on developing body awareness during movement. Chapter 5 discusses the anatomy and biomechanics related to Pilates exercise. Chapter 6 details all of the Pilates exercises included in the YMCA program, and it includes suggested formats for different levels of classes. Chapter 7 concludes the book with information on teaching skills that will help the YMCA Pilates instructor be successful. The appendix provides useful information and resources for your YMCA Pilates program.

There is growing scientific evidence that certain types of mind–body exercise promote improvements in health. And, mind–body exercise programs such as Pilates are consistent with the mission statement of the YMCA movement: to put Christian principles into practice through programs that build a healthy spirit, mind, and body for all. These programs are also consistent with the eight goals outlined in the YMCA constitution, especially the fourth: "To appreciate that health of mind and body is a sacred gift and that physical fitness and mental well-being are conditions to be achieved and maintained." (For the complete set of goals, go to www.ymca.net.)

The popularity of Pilates exercise today means that many communities probably have a significant number of people who already practice this form of exercise, have tried it at home with a video, or are interested in starting. By offering this program, YMCAs have the opportunity to reach a number of people who may not be interested in traditional exercise, but who may come to the YMCA to experience Pilates. Because the YMCA Pilates program is flexible, it can enhance almost any YMCA's program offerings. See what it can do for yours.

Acknowledgments

YMCA of the USA would like to acknowledge the contributions of those individuals who helped in the development of the *YMCA Pilates Instructor Manual:*

Consultant and Writer
Adita Yrizarry, Professional Fitness, Inc. Key Biscayne, FL. Web site: www.professional-fitness.com

Project Coordinator and Manual Editor
Michael J. Spezzano, Specialty Consultant for Health and Fitness, YMCA of the USA, Chicago, IL

Editorial Reviewers
Celeste Wroblewski, former Director, Knowledge Publishing & Products, YMCA of the USA, Chicago, IL

Elizabeth Fleck, Editorial Specialist, Knowledge Publishing & Products, YMCA of the USA, Chicago, IL

Donna Fisher, Pilates Director, Cooper Fitness Center, Dallas, TX

Exercise models
Miki Dagan
Adita Yrizarry

Wardrobe
Couture Active Wear

YMCA of the USA would also like to gratefully acknowledge the contributions and cooperation received from the International Sports Conditioning Association and Thomas "The Promise" Trebotich in the development of this manual and the accompanying training course for YMCA instructors.

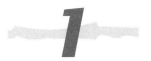

The YMCA Pilates Program

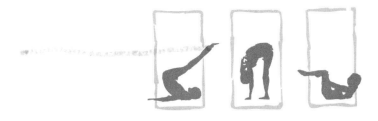

YMCA Pilates is an entry-level Pilates mat exercise program that YMCAs can use to introduce Pilates to their members and to other people in their communities. YMCA of the USA developed it in collaboration with Pilates program experts. This manual and the accompanying instructor certification course available from YMCA of the USA are designed to educate YMCA health and fitness instructors about the benefits and techniques of Pilates exercise and to equip those instructors with the tools to begin a Pilates mat exercise program at their YMCA.

The YMCA is recognized as a leader in promoting health and fitness in communities across the nation. YMCAs collectively are the largest nonprofit community service organization in America, and they have a long history of developing and implementing programs that help people develop in spirit, mind, and body. YMCA programs meet the health, recreation, and social needs of nearly 19 million children, teens, and adults. Maintaining regular physical activity is key to achieving a healthful lifestyle because it decreases the risk of developing many health-related problems including heart disease, high blood pressure, diabetes, and joint disease.

For more than 100 years, the YMCA movement has embraced a holistic philosophy that is based on integrating spirit, mind, and body. Today, leaders in the health and fitness industry are increasingly recognizing the value of integrating these three elements into exercise programs. Since the early 1990s, exercise programs such as Pilates, yoga, and tai chi have become characterized as *mind–body* programs, and have risen dramatically in popularity. YMCAs, along with other health and fitness providers, are responding accordingly to member requests to add these programs to their activities and services. YMCA of the USA uses the definition of mind–body exercise developed in 1997 by the IDEA Mind–Body Fitness Committee: "physical exercise executed with a profound inwardly directed focus" (Carrico 1996, p.42). Mind–body exercise includes these characteristics:

- Inner mental focus
- Concentration on muscular movements
- Synchronization of movements with breathing patterns
- Attention to form and alignment

In recent years, the range of mind–body exercise programs has diversified and expanded to include traditional methods that have evolved from ancient times as well as modern adaptations that teach movement grounded in science. Some of the variations seen today are truly a mix of the old and the new, such as programs combining cardiovascular exercise with a quiet, focused component. Yoga and Pilates are two of the more popular forms of mind–body exercise practiced today. Although some similarities exist between the two forms, yoga is a 5,000-year-old ancient art that requires moving from one static posture to the next without repetition, while Pilates is a more modern exercise method involving a series of flowing movements that are more dynamic.

The current popularity of Pilates exercise started in the 1970s, grew steadily through the 1980s, and virtually exploded during the 1990s. The number of dedicated Pilates studios has grown from just five worldwide in 1976 to over 5,000 in 2003. Celebrities and professional athletes have become attracted to this form of exercise, undoubtedly fueling its growth. Researchers estimate that 2.4 million Americans practice Pilates (SGMA International 2002). For a largely inactive American population, adhering to any form of regular physical activity has been a difficult process. There may be many reasons for this, but attempts at regular exercise have been discouraging to many. Pilates exercise offers some hope to frustrated would-be exercisers, because mind–body programs such as Pilates may be more appealing than more conventional exercise programs. Some people speculate that the self-directed focus and reduced intensity of mind–body exercise may be factors in improving participant motivation and adherence to exercise. Because mind–body exercise provides so many health benefits, people could make long-term improvements in their health by adopting and adhering to programs of this nature.

Benefits of Pilates Exercise

The YMCA Pilates exercise program offers local YMCAs a new option for their health and fitness programs, in particular, one that will help reach those people who might not become involved in other forms of exercise. Although some YMCAs have offered Pilates and other mind–body exercise programs in the past, this new program offers a standard format and a simple way for many YMCAs to begin offering it at minimal cost. YMCA members will be able to experience many benefits by participating in YMCA Pilates exercise, including the following:

- **Core muscle development:** Maintaining a constant focus on trunk stability throughout the workout strengthens abdominal and back muscles.
- **Improved posture:** Restoring the body's natural alignment leads to better posture in all situations.
- **Injury prevention:** Improving muscular control and balance helps to prevent injuries that commonly occur during impact exercises and daily tasks.
- **Relief of stress and tension:** Practicing focused breathing and concentration during exercise helps to tune out other distractions, producing a revitalizing effect.
- **Enhanced body awareness:** Focusing on the body's movement and learning to move more efficiently during exercise result in using the body more efficiently throughout the day.
- **Balance of strength and flexibility:** Developing muscles around joints that are balanced in strength and flexibility enables them to work effectively and reduces their risk of injury.
- **Enhanced athletic performance:** Participating regularly in Pilates exercise enhances performance in lifetime sports such as golf, tennis, skating, and many others.
- **Increased self-esteem:** Learning to successfully perform Pilates exercises and seeing the results of the effort boost feelings of accomplishment and self-worth.

- Mental Focus
- increase balance & control

Beginning a Pilates Exercise Program

One of the advantages of Pilates exercise is its adaptability: You can offer it in a number of formats, depending on the YMCA's capabilities and the community's needs. Pilates exercise can reach a wide range of participants, from young to old and from beginner to elite athletes. The YMCA's challenge is to design a program that accommodates all participants' skill and fitness levels and meets their individual needs. Meeting this challenge requires not only that instructors be trained and skillful in teaching Pilates exercise but also that the organization be committed to successfully implementing the program. Given the current popularity of Pilates, many members are probably asking for a program, and other community organizations are likely offering one. Because Pilates has the impressive list of benefits just detailed, many YMCAs will want to respond to these requests and offer the program. Doing so, however, will require some research, planning, and training to ensure a quality program.

Before beginning a Pilates program, YMCA staff need to understand that mind–body programs differ philosophically and practically from more physically focused fitness modalities such as step aerobics or group cycling. High-energy movements during which participants mimic the instructor, accompanied by music with a loud, driving beat, often characterize traditional exercise programs. In these programs, usually little attention is given to precision of movement and body alignment. Pilates is not simply a series of exercises to be performed; it is a mind–body discipline that combines core stabilization and mobility training for improving the body's function. In this regard, Pilates is a relatively complex activity compared to many traditional exercise formats. There are more than 500 different Pilates exercises and variations. Many of these exercises can be performed on either a mat or specialized pieces of equipment, or both. Facilities offering Pilates have to make several implementation decisions such as whether to offer group classes or individual sessions and whether to offer mat- or equipment-based classes. The YMCA Pilates program provides an entry-level program that is relatively easy to implement and build on once successfully launched.

Program Options

The large number of exercises and wide variety of class formats available will allow YMCAs to develop Pilates exercise programs with almost any budget. In the basic program presented in this manual and accompanying certification course, the only equipment required is an exercise mat for each participant. Group mat classes provide an easy, low-risk, and inexpensive way for YMCAs to begin Pilates programming while participants' interest and instructors' organizational experience grow. Although the scope of the YMCA program and this manual is limited to mat exercise programs for groups, and the optional use of small equipment such as resistance bands and rings, YMCAs may graduate to offering programs with larger equipment such as the Reformer, which is used primarily for individual work. Such additions increase the variety of exercises and the options for participants who continue in the program, but they also increase expenses for the YMCA.

Mat-Based Classes

Pilates mat classes focus on developing core muscle stability and learning the basic biomechanical principles of Pilates. To launch a program, many facilities will offer a few introductory sessions for members and other new participants. These sessions typically generate enough interest to warrant conducting regular Pilates classes.

Depending on time and facility availability, plan on offering at least one hour-long class that meets two or three times a week. You can add more sessions as interest and demand grow. A typical exercise studio of about 1,000 square feet makes a good environment for a Pilates mat class. In addition to requiring individual exercise mats, some group classes can use small pieces of exercise equipment such as rings or bands for resistance.

Equipment-Based Sessions

The two largest pieces of Pilates exercise equipment are the Cadillac and the Reformer, both of which include padded benches with frames of pulleys and cables. This equipment can be expensive to purchase, and it will require dedicated program space. Therefore, the decision to implement equipment-based programs is a significant one, which is why we recommend beginning with a mat program format in your YMCA. Unlike mat classes, equipment-based Pilates is usually conducted in a one-on-one format similar to personal training, or it is conducted in small groups of four to eight participants. This personal attention allows the instructor to individualize the workout for maximum effectiveness, and it may provide additional motivation to the participant. You can start an equipment-based program with as little as one Reformer, which costs approximately $2,500. Although this initial purchase can seem relatively modest, you generally should not consider implementing equipment-based programs unless your YMCA is prepared to dedicate a room of at least 600 square feet specifically to Pilates equipment.

Pilates As a YMCA Program

As with all YMCA programs, you should offer Pilates at your YMCA in a way that is consistent with the mission, goals, and values of the YMCA movement.

YMCA Mission

The mission statement of the YMCA movement is "to put Christian principles into practice through programs that build healthy spirit, mind, and body for all." Your YMCA may have a slightly different statement, but it is probably very similar to this one. If you don't know what your YMCA's mission statement is, ask someone who does.

YMCA Goals

In the 1970s, the National Council of YMCAs (to which all YMCAs in the United States belong) created eight goals and published them in the preamble to its constitution and bylaws. The preamble states that the goals are for "our members and their constituents," in other words, local YMCAs and the children, teens, and adults they serve and involve. All YMCA programs, activities, and endeavors, including YMCA Pilates, should help people to develop and enhance each of the characteristics and behaviors outlined in the list that follows. Note that the words in **bold** are contemporary summaries of each goal; they are not published in the constitution. Also, some YMCAs have adopted goal statements that are worded differently from these, but they are effectively similar.

YMCAs build healthy spirit, mind, and body by helping people develop the following:

1. **Self-worth:** To develop self-confidence and self-respect and an appreciation of their own worth as individuals.
2. **Christian principles:** To develop a faith for daily living based on the teachings of Jesus Christ, that they may thereby be helped in achieving their highest potential as children of God.
3. **Positive relationships:** To grow as responsible members of their families and citizens of their communities.
4. **Holistic health:** To appreciate that health of mind and body is a sacred gift and that physical fitness and mental well-being are conditions to be achieved and maintained.
5. **Appreciation of diversity:** To recognize the worth of all persons and to work for interracial and intergroup understanding.
6. **International awareness:** To develop a sense of world-mindedness and to work for worldwide understanding.
7. **Leadership and service:** To develop their capacities for leadership and use them

responsibly in their own groups and in community life.

8. **Environmental stewardship:** To appreciate the beauty, diversity, and interdependence of all forms of life and all resources that God has provided in this world and to develop an ethical basis for guiding the relationships of mankind with the rest of God's natural community.

YMCA Values

Four core values guide YMCAs in pursuing the YMCA mission and goals. YMCA of the USA adopted them in the 1990s as part of a recommitment to character development. Many YMCAs have adopted the four core values in the list that follows, but some may have a slightly different or expanded list. Some YMCAs consider these values to be an expression of the Christian principles referenced in both the mission statement and contemporary summaries of the goals (listed in the previous section). These values are both practiced in operations and promoted in all programs, including Pilates:

- **Caring:** To demonstrate a sincere concern for others, for their needs and well-being.
- **Honesty:** To tell the truth and to demonstrate reliability and trustworthiness through actions that are in keeping with your stated positions and beliefs.
- **Respect:** To treat others as you would want them to treat you; to value the worth of every person, including yourself.
- **Responsibility:** To do what is right, what you ought to do; to be accountable for your promises and your choices of behavior and actions.

* when ever a muscle contracts the opposing muscle stretches

* Use breath w/movement, Most important is to breath.

2

Introduction to Pilates

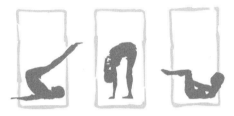

The health and fitness movement in the United States has been inundated with a variety of exercise programs, routines, philosophies, and equipment that promise to develop physical fitness. Some focus on a specific component of fitness, some use specific types of equipment, and some have questionable value. In the early 1900s, Joseph H. Pilates developed a unique system of stretching and strengthening exercises designed to work the body as a whole, focusing on the abdominal, lower back, and gluteal muscles. In the United States, this form of exercise became tremendously popular with ballet dancers, who quickly embraced its practice and philosophy; but the Pilates Method did not move beyond this relatively small circle into the mainstream for many years.

During the American fitness boom of the late 20th century, programs and equipment that were designed to improve cardiovascular conditioning and muscular strength were the most popular forms of exercise. As more people tried various exercise routines, exercise-related injuries became all too common, largely because of factors including overuse, poor body alignment, improper form, and an aging participant population. Many turned to more natural exercises that would make the body functionally stronger and more flexible, including older

forms of exercise such as yoga and other forms. In addition to being gentler, these exercises took a more holistic approach to improving physical fitness of spirit, mind, and body. As part of this movement, Pilates exercise has made a remarkable resurgence and is now more popular than ever.

Pilates exercise was developed around the principle of moving the body as a whole, recognizing that every muscle in the body is meant to work in conjunction with an array of neighboring muscles. In everyday movements of the human body, no muscle acts entirely on its own; muscles work in unison, each contributing a certain percentage of the total effort. However, many exercise programs focus only on specific muscle groups. This narrow focus can create imbalances in body development and structure and can often lead to injury. Pilates works on creating balance in the human structure through purposeful movement, body awareness, and focused breathing.

As part of this acceptance of mind-body programs, fitness practitioners have embraced the concept of core conditioning, exercise designed to strengthen the core, or trunk, of the body—the abdomen, the pelvis, and the back. Years ago, Joseph Pilates recognized the need to address this area, which he referred to

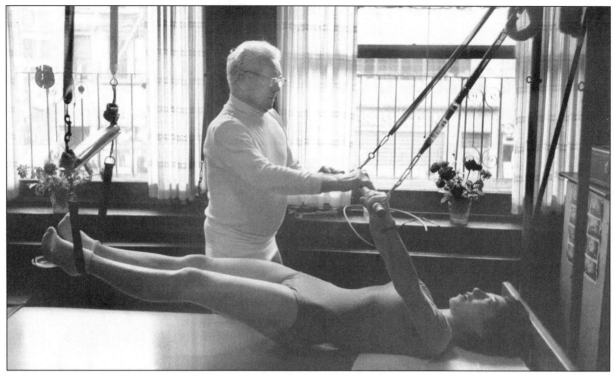

Joseph Pilates working with a client on the Cadillac.

as the *powerhouse* of the body. Pilates realized long ago that a strong, flexible core musculature enables the body to function more efficiently, avoid injury, and enjoy balanced movement.

The Pilates Method

Joseph Pilates referred to his Method as *Contrology*, a balanced approach to strengthening and stretching the body in a mindful manner. Performing Pilates movements correctly requires concentration, proper posture, and fluid breathing to have positive effects on the body. To minimize stress to the body from the gravitational forces occurring during standing exercise, Pilates movements are primarily performed lying down or seated. An array of specialized devices and props can also be used for variety and to enhance training.

The Pilates Method includes the following programming and equipment options:

• **Pilates mat exercise:** This is a series of exercises that are performed on a floor mat using few or no props and whose movements develop muscular strength and flexibility. Joseph Pilates' original method of Contrology

consisted of mat exercise with no equipment. The YMCA Pilates Program is a basic version of Pilates mat exercises.

• **Pilates equipment exercise using the Cadillac:** Initially designed for rehabilitation of bed-ridden patients, this device consists of a flat bench on a frame, roughly the size of a bed, with an intricate array of springs and pulleys attached to it (see figure 2.1a). These pulleys apply resistance and also assist the participant in performing movements to strengthen the core muscles with little to no impact on the joints.

• **Pilates equipment exercise using the Reformer:** The Reformer is a device similar to the Cadillac, but it has a bed that slides back and forth, is usually more compact, and is without a frame overhead (see figure 2.1b). The movable bed on the Reformer creates different body positions and angles from which the participant can perform a wider array of exercises than those performed on the Cadillac.

• **Exercise props:** These devices can be incorporated into mat exercise programs for specialized training and to address individual

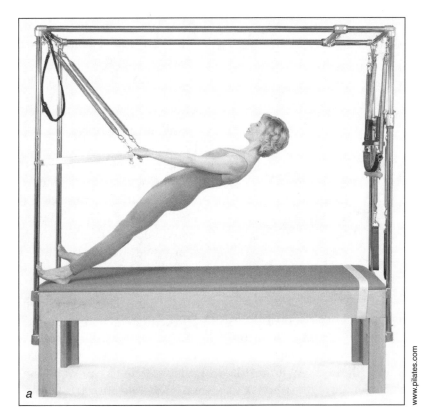

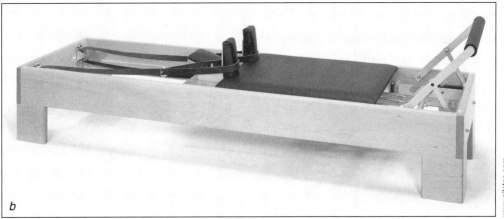

Figure 2.1 *(a)* The Cadillac machine. *(b)* The Reformer machine.

participants' needs (see figure 2.2). Exercise props include the following:

- **Resistance band:** a flat elastic band used to provide resistance to movement as well as enhance stability
- **Magic Circle:** a round, spring steel or plastic ring with handles
- **Stability ball:** a large, inflatable rubber or plastic ball commonly used in exercise programs

The Life of Joseph Pilates

Joseph H. Pilates was born in Germany in 1880. As a child he suffered from asthma and rickets (underdevelopment in cartilage and new bone due to a vitamin D deficiency), which set him on a lifelong search for ways to improve his physique and endurance. After discovering that exercise was an effective way to manage his health, he made it a way of life. A constant

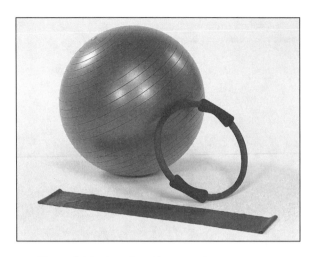

Figure 2.2 Props often used in Pilates mat exercise programs.

student of human movement, Joseph Pilates included bodybuilding, gymnastics, boxing, and yoga in his workout routine, later to be refined into the Pilates Method. As an adult, he worked as a circus acrobat and a boxer in England. During World War I, he was interned with other German nationals living in England. Because of his compelling desire and need to continue exercising, Joseph Pilates practiced his series of strength and flexibility exercises even in limited living quarters. Other prisoners became curious about his daily exercise regimen, and he began to teach it to them.

The British military soon became aware of

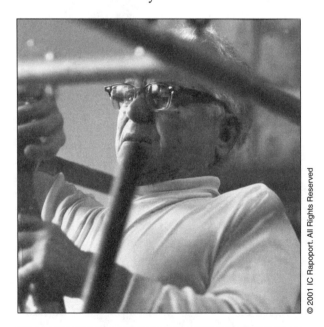

Joseph Pilates, the inventor of Pilates exercise.

this unique training program, which was keeping groups of prisoners healthier than others and immune to an epidemic of influenza. They soon removed Joseph Pilates from his barracks and put him to work as a rehabilitation nurse in the camp hospital. Believing that movement would improve circulation, avoid atrophy, and lead to healing of injuries, he devised a way to help bed-ridden patients to move. By placing springs and pulleys on their beds to assist injured soldiers in moving their limbs, he created the forerunner of the future Cadillac exercise device. Through Joseph Pilates' methods, many war victims became strong and well.

In 1926, Joseph Pilates embarked on a voyage to New York City, during which he met his future wife, Clara. They soon opened the first Pilates Studio there, which happened to be located next to a ballet school. His form of exercise became very popular in the dance community. Dancers praised it for its ease of movement and emphasis on postural control. Pilates claimed that "In ten sessions, you will feel the difference. In twenty, you will see the difference, and in thirty, you'll have a whole new body" (Gallagher and Kryzanowowska 2000, p. 23). Pilates soon developed a reputation for relieving pain and increasing strength and flexibility through his unique exercise regime. Although primarily confined to the dance and athletic communities, he nonetheless enjoyed a devout, if small, following for years. By 1945, he wrote his first book, *Return to Life Through Contrology,* and proceeded to train instructors to follow in his method. He maintained the highest level of personal physical fitness throughout his life. In 1967, at the age of 87, Joseph H. Pilates died of smoke inhalation in a shed fire. After his death, Clara continued his legacy and joined forces with protégé Romana Kryzanowowska to build the Pilates program that is known today.

In his book *Return to Life Through Contrology,* Joseph Pilates defined physical fitness in the following manner: "Physical fitness is the first requisite to happiness. Our interpretation of physical fitness is the attainment and maintenance of a uniformly developed body with sound mind fully capable of naturally, easily, and satisfactorily performing our many and varied daily tasks with spontaneous zest and pleasure" (Pilates and Miller 1998, p. 6).

3

Philosophy of Pilates Mat Work

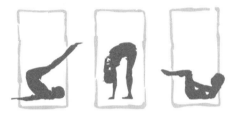

Pilates mat work is a series of movements that flow from one to the other, causing muscle groups to strengthen and stretch according to their biomechanical needs. The program is designed to initially undo years of poor habits by reteaching the body to move, focusing the mind on purposeful movement, creating muscular balance, and improving posture. Pilates has a core selection of exercises with hundreds of possible variations used for creating a workout or routine. All of them have names and involve dynamic movement, as opposed to many yoga postures, which are static. *Progression* in Pilates exercise does not necessarily mean doing more or advanced exercise; it involves mastery and continued practice of focused movement.

The guiding tenet behind Pilates exercise is the biomechanical principle that whenever a muscle contracts, its opposing muscle stretches. When muscles contract and pull on the bones to which they are attached, body movement is created. This pulling is not the result of one muscle working alone but rather is a coordinated effort from a group of muscles working in unison, with various degrees of force, resulting in movement in a specific direction. Each muscle in the group is responsible for a specific percentage of the work; when any muscle in the

group is too strong, too weak, too tight, or too loose, imbalances occur. Over time, muscular imbalances can lead to injury.

Postural Enhancement

Joseph Pilates concentrated his efforts on the *powerhouse*, or core, of the body, because creating a strong core stabilizes the spine and creates a redefined posture for the body. When the core of the body achieves strength and postural alignment, the entire body becomes stronger, movement becomes fluid, and injuries are less common. Pilates mat work is designed to teach the body to correctly perform movements that are required in daily activity. As program participants adopt new habits for strengthening the body's core and become more mindful of their movements, the body will eventually adopt new, more efficient ways of sitting, standing, and performing activities. With proper postural alignment and strength, the spine will actually expand and elongate, allowing the participants to assume their natural height.

A benefit of this emphasis on posture is that the muscles known as the *stabilizers* will become stronger. These are the small groups of muscles that are responsible for maintaining the integrity of joints. Once these muscles have become stronger, they can work together with the primary muscles to create a strong, flexible, properly aligned body (see figure 3.1).

The Mind–Body Connection

Unless trained to engage the mind during movement, people will tend to focus on one area of the body or one aspect of the movement without incorporating the mind and the rest of the body in the process. Pilates mat work teaches participants to use the mind–body connection to create purposeful movement.

Traditional fitness programs typically teach participants to follow an instructor through a particular routine, with the only focus being to perform a movement in what they perceive to be the correct manner. Joseph Pilates believed that movement had to be exact and mindful—that the mind worked together with the muscles to create both physical and mental health. It is one thing to simply perform a movement; it is another to understand all aspects of that movement and perform it in a conscious, controlled manner. As a Pilates mat exercise instructor, you should teach movements with proper biomechanics and breathing techniques so that the participants will understand the various components of each movement and so that they can make the movements flow naturally from one phase to another. In addition, you should teach participants to have full recognition of their exercise form and to modify and correct their own techniques without comparing themselves to others. Each participant in Pilates exercise should recognize their own unique facets of movement and create a natural flow with each movement they make.

Breathing and Movement

Breathing affects all the functions of the body, because each cell in the body requires oxygen to perform its duties. Incorporating the breath in unison with the movement helps participants focus and pay closer attention to what they are doing, creating what has been termed a *mindful approach* to exercise, eliminating the day-to-day chatter of the mind, calming the body as a whole, and relieving stress. When a participant grasps the connection of the mind and the body, the two parts can positively affect each other: The mind trains the body to eliminate improper form and technique through improved skill and repetition, and it utilizes the flow of oxygen for muscular nourishment and mental clarity. Focused breathing during Pilates exercise has two applications:

1. It helps to create a rhythm for movement and to focus concentration of effort. If used correctly, the breath can become hypnotic. When enough concentration is placed on the breath, the mind is diverted from focusing on the day's

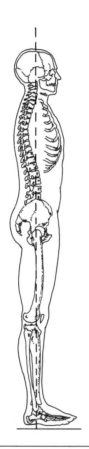

Figure 3.1 Side view of ideal alignment.

Reprinted, by permission, from J.C. Griffin, 1998, *Client-centered exercise prescription.* (Champaign, IL: Human Kinetics), 66.

events. This gives the mind a chance to slow down and to relax. In addition, the coordination of breath with movement can help movement become more fluid, as the mind focuses on what the body is doing.

2. It helps to cleanse the body internally. Each inhalation brings in oxygen to help fuel and nourish the body, and each exhalation removes waste products out of the system.

Beginning Pilates participants are often conspicuous about the noise they may make when breathing deeply. The section on breathing in chapter 4 (see pages 17-18) will help you learn to teach participants to overcome this self-consciousness and not to worry if they cannot exactly match the breathing pattern with the movement. You fully appreciate and understand the impact of breathing and its relationship to movement in order to teach this concept to your participants.

4

Kinesthetic Awareness

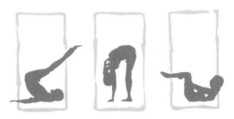

Kinesthetic awareness is the ability to know exactly where the body is in space—how the body is positioned during movement, how it should move most effectively and efficiently, and how it should feel during that movement. Teaching this concept is a significant challenge. You must continually point out that participants need to be conscious of every movement; this repetition and heightened awareness breed accomplishment. You can help participants master kinesthetic awareness by giving accurate, specific verbal cues to describe the desired movement and to give corrective tips.

For example, when teaching an abdominal crunch, you might tell participants to place both hands behind the head and pull the abdominal muscles in while crunching up. This is how most instructors describe the movement (see figure 4.1a). However, in reality the abdominal muscles run from the ribs to the pelvis, and the desired execution of the movement is to draw the rib cage in and down toward the pelvis, which in turn lifts the upper body off the floor. By providing specific directions and calling participants' attention to the correct movement, you will train them to focus on what they are doing, eventually resulting in more efficient movement (see figure 4.1b).

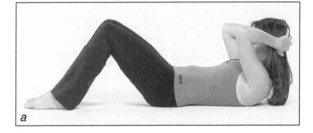

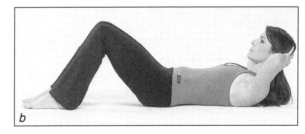

Figure 4.1 *(a)* Incorrect crunch position. *(b)* Correct crunch position.

The average exercise class participant does not focus on feeling the muscular contraction during movement. One of the primary principles in Pilates is to concentrate on this feeling and make precise movements. In his book *Return to Life Through Contrology*, Joseph Pilates said, "Ideally, our muscles should obey our will. Reasonably, our will should not be dominated by reflex actions of our muscles" (Pilates and Miller 1998, p. 10). In typical fitness regimes, instructors only teach participants to perform certain exercises for a particular goal (for example, endurance, strength, or flexibility) without teaching the principles of biomechanics and muscular contraction to help them perform the movement more efficiently and effectively. Joseph Pilates called this *mindless exercise* and preached a more mindful control of movement, leading to both physical and mental well-being.

Instructors of traditional exercise classes often train participants to focus on what the instructor is doing, instead of focusing on what they feel. As a Pilates instructor, you will teach participants how to visualize a movement in the mind, how to move to accomplish it, and then how to feel if the body is in the correct position. Once participants are fully aware of the body placement and positioning in space, they can effectively stabilize the body in the correct position. In order for them to receive the full benefit of a movement, you should teach your Pilates participants to understand the motion in such a complete way that they can feel any misalignments or discrepancies and make the required technique corrections. Once you help them achieve this awareness, they will progress quite rapidly.

In the course of daily life, the human body moves instinctively as a whole. Without a lot of thought, the body can run, jump, climb, and pick things up, using an array of muscles for a variety of intricate movements. For example, the body is fully aware that, in order to walk, one leg must go in front of the other and the feet should face in the direction of movement. The mind doesn't need to instruct the body to do this; the natural flow of movement made possible by muscles working together is the way the body was designed to move. Sometimes when we perform activites of daily living or some form of exercise we focus on using only an isolated muscle, and this principle is lost, and isolated rather than coordinated muscular action takes over. Unfortunately, with years of isolated movements, the body develops poor alignment, poor posture, and muscle imbalances. For example, the hips become misaligned, or there is pain in a particular area of the leg, leaving one leg to work harder than

the other. Without recognition and correction, these imbalances worsen and create additional structural imbalances (see figure 4.2). The more aware people become of their movements, the greater the chance that they will be able to correct imbalances and reduce the incidence of further pain or discomfort.

In order for you to teach the concept of kinesthetic awareness, you first need to develop it yourself. Hours of individual work on the exercises will help you recognize your own physical imbalances and work to correct them. The more you work on your own technique, the easier it will be to teach the exercises in a way that participants will clearly understand them. Because of the precise nature of Pilates exercise, only trained and certified instructors should teach a Pilates class.

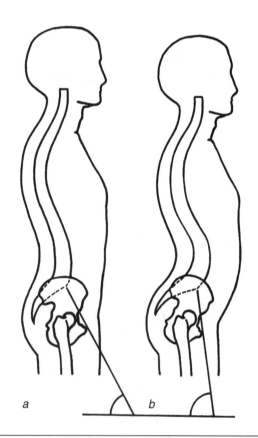

Figure 4.2 *(a)* Proper alignment as a result of movement awareness. *(b)* Misalignment in the hips as a result of years of imbalanced movement.

Reprinted, by permission, from J. Watkins, 1999, *Structure and function of the musculoskeletal* system. (Champaign, IL: Human Kinetics), 167.

Movement and Muscular Control

Unconscious movement is not a challenge for a human being; we can move with virtually no thought involved. The challenge becomes to move with full awareness of the muscles' contracting and having the ability to control the movement. In Pilates, this focus must start with the core musculature of the trunk, the body's powerhouse. To see how this basic Pilates concept applies to everyday life, consider an untrained person sitting in a chair in a mindless manner, slouching and sinking into the chair. The effect of Pilates training on daily life will be that the same person will be more conscious of this simple task and perform the movement mindfully—sitting from the base of the spine and then elongating the spine. Slouching promotes incorrect posture, lower back soreness, and abdominal protrusion. Pilates teaches participants to initiate all movement at the core and maintain an elongated spine during movement, causing the abdominal muscles and back to work together as a team.

Joseph Pilates wanted people to use the mind to take full charge of the body during movement. A basic premise of Pilates exercise is that, once trained to think and move in this manner, the body will be able to feel areas of misalignment and correct itself from within. A Pilates exercise program teaches participants not to focus just on the part of the body performing the movement but to broaden the focus to include all the surrounding areas of the body. This practice helps to create a unity of all the areas working together rather than a situation of individual muscles working in isolation. For example, consider what the body must do to correctly perform the simple push-up exercise. Initially, the exerciser focuses attention on the work of the arms lowering the body. But when the exerciser considers the whole body, the focus expands to include the muscles that stabilize the body's core, the legs, the shoulders, and the arms and chest. All of this muscular activation creates a stable body with muscle groups working together to correctly perform the movement. You must develop a sharp eye for observing and analyzing movement to draw participants' attention to specific areas that may not be activated when they should be.

Precision of Movement

As a Pilates instructor, you are expected to teach, review, analyze, and repeat all movements so that participants will feel confident about their technique. Once participants understand a movement and the related body placement and technique, they can begin to move with greater precision. Participants will invariably lose precise control of technique when they are distracted mentally or physically and lose focus. Besides creating inefficiency of movement, it is interesting to note that poor technique, not the movement per se, is often what leads to injury.

When the mind wanders, the body usually loses its focus on performing precise movement. You must continually observe technique and teach precision of each movement as constant reminders for participants to be aware of their bodies. To accomplish this awareness, you will need to give more personalized attention and direction than in a traditional group exercise class because everyone's body and movements are unique. Participants' technique and effort will be inspired and motivated by what you say and how you say it, as well as by your praise and support for their accomplishments. Remember that Pilates is meant to meet each participant's individual needs, so you must encourage each of your participants to work within their own means, not try to compete with nor compare themselves to others.

The Role of Focused Breathing

In Pilates exercise, focused breathing is crucial in helping to refocus the mind when it has decided to disengage itself from the movement. Every participant has the power to improve technique by placing concentrated energy into the movement and into the breath. Joseph Pilates embraced the notion that breathing was a form of invigoration and power. Focused breathing also helps to alleviate stress during exercise and expand the lungs. The lungs are

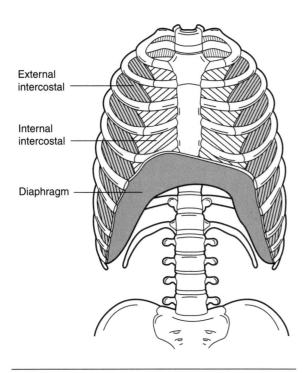

External
intercostal

Internal
intercostal

Diaphragm

Figure 4.3 Anterior view of main respiratory muscles.

Reprinted, by permission, from R.S. Behnke, 2001, *Kinetic anatomy.* (Champaign, IL: Human Kinetics), 163.

encased in the thoracic cavity of the rib cage, with the diaphragm sitting at the base of the lungs (see figure 4.3). Deep breathing during Pilates exercise increases the amount of oxygen into the lungs in two ways:

1. The rib cage expands, thus allowing more oxygen to enter the lungs.

2. The diaphragm contracts and pulls the dome of the lungs downward, enabling more air to enter.

The respiratory system is controlled by the autonomic nervous system, meaning that the act of breathing is unconscious and automatic. Dealing with daily stress, rushing, meditating, and exercising all change the rate of breath. However, breathing patterns can be controlled consciously. For example, when a person becomes angry or anxious, their breathing typically becomes shallow and rapid. A more mindful approach to breathing can slow down the breath rate and increase the amount of oxygen coming into the lungs, naturally slowing the heart rate, relaxing the mind, and calming the body.

Because Pilates is designed to be a complete form of exercise for the human body, breathing is an essential part of the discipline. With each Pilates movement performed, there is a corresponding breathing pattern. You should teach these movements and breathing slowly to encourage a deeper inspiration and expiration of air, keeping the focus on the movement and eliminating other thoughts and physical distractions. You will learn the details of how to employ correct breathing technique without compromising the body's core musculature in the next chapter.

5

Anatomy and Biomechanics

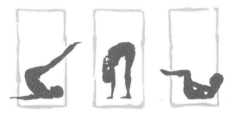

As a Pilates exercise instructor, you should study human anatomy, particularly so that you can understand how the structure of the body relates to the function of the exercise. In other words, it will be useful for you to know the practical application of the body's musculo-skeletal system. The information in this chapter should supplement your existing knowledge of anatomy and biomechanics, serve as additional information and review on the subjects, and describe how they relate to Pilates exercise. The more you understand about movement and anatomy, the more effective you will be as a Pilates instructor.

Functional Anatomy

The musculoskeletal system of the body is composed of an intricate web of muscles, tendons, ligaments, and bones. Depending on the movement being performed, these components can act as initiators, stabilizers, and primary movers of the body. Movement will produce action at one or more of the body's joints. Each joint has a range of motion (ROM) that is specific to that joint and is dictated by

- the type and structure of the joint;

- any bones and bony surfaces around the joint; and

- any muscles, tendons, and ligaments related to the joint.

Joint ROM can be compromised if the surrounding stabilizer muscles are not working in concert with the primary mover muscle. As a result, the joints could have restricted mobility or, conversely, excessive ROM and laxity. In addition, if one of the stabilizing muscles is stronger than the rest, the imbalance can cause instability. Many muscular injuries occur when such an imbalance exists.

To visualize this situation, consider a game of tug-of-war: If you have two teams of equal strengths on each side of the rope, the rope doesn't move and you have a stable situation. However, if one team is stronger than the other, the stronger team will pull harder and pull the weaker team, resulting in instability.

The muscles of the human body were designed to work together as a team in producing movement and maintaining structural integrity. The effects of time and the repetition of poor habits often have undesirable effects on the body's structure and function, such as joint instability or muscular imbalance. For example, when children walk, they will unconsciously hold the head up, lift the chest, and pull the shoulders back. Over time, perhaps because of stress, work, or inactivity, the typical adult lets the head come forward and rounds the shoulders, which can lead to poor posture and an abnormal curvature of the spine. This poor posture will then have detrimental effects throughout the body, creating stress and imbalances in the lower back, hips, knees, and ankles with a domino-like effect. The following section describes three conditions that commonly result from misalignment and poor posture.

✳ Common Postural Misalignments

To teach a successful Pilates program, you should understand the effects of postural misalignments because, if present, they will effect the form and technique of participants when performing many Pilates exercises. The three most common postural misalignments are:

• **Upper cross syndrome:** This condition occurs when the head and shoulders come forward, causing an increase in the curvature of the upper portion of the spine. It leads to tightness in the anterior muscles of the upper trunk, the pectoralis major and minor, sternocleidomastoid, upper trapezius, and levator scapulae muscles. In addition, the condition causes weakness in the posterior muscles of the upper trunk, the rhomboids, deep neck flexors, middle and lower trapezius, and serratus anterior musculature (see figure 5.1a).

• **Lower cross syndrome:** This condition is characterized by an increased forward curve of the lower back, which causes the abdomen in front and gluteals in back to protrude outward. This condition leads to tightness in the posterior muscles of the lower trunk, the lumbar erector spinae, and the psoas major. In addition, the anterior muscles of the lower trunk, rectus abdominis, external obliques, and gluteus maximus become weak and do not effectively support the body in proper postural alignment (see figure 5.1b).

• **Flat back syndrome:** This condition is a decrease of the natural curvature of the lower back, resulting in a back that appears flat when viewed from the side, rather than curved. The hamstrings and rectus abdominis muscles become excessively tight, and the hip flexors and lumbar erector spinae become weak (see figure 5.1c).

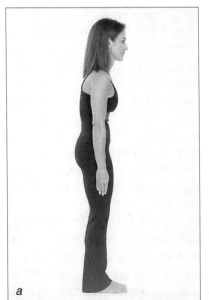 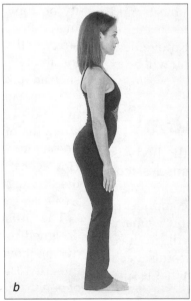 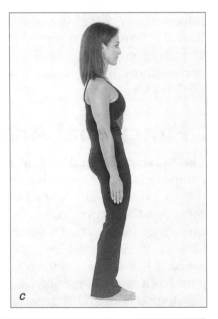

Figure 5.1 Syndromes caused by poor posture and misalignment include (a) upper cross syndrome, (b) lower cross syndrome, and (c) flat back syndrome.

An important goal of any exercise program should be to achieve muscular balance, because the syndromes just described often result from imbalances in muscular strength and flexibility. Most muscular imbalances occur as a result of continued poor posture over several years and the repetition of movements that create the imbalance. Regular practice of Pilates exercise can dramatically improve these postural misalignment syndromes. One of the often-quoted claims made by Joseph Pilates was that his Contrology program had the ability to add inches to one's stature (Pilates and Miller 1998, p. 17). Although practicing Pilates exercise will not technically cause a person to grow, retraining the spine and musculature can make a person stand taller and in a proper, more natural alignment. This retraining can develop the body in such a way that the person's posture improves and stature increases.

Muscular Anatomy

A practical understanding of muscular anatomy for Pilates instructors involves knowing all the muscles involved in the body's major joint actions. Figures 5.2 through 5.7 on pages 22 to 27 detail the following muscles of the shoulder, elbow, hip, knee and ankle joints (muscle actions follow in parentheses).

- Shoulder joint
  - Deltoid (abduction; anterior fibers: flexion, internal rotation; posterior fibers: extension, external rotation)
  - Pectoralis major (flexion, adduction, internal rotation)
  - Latissimus dorsi (extension adduction, internal rotation)
- Elbow joint
  - Triceps brachii (extension)
  - Biceps brachii (flexion, forearm supination)
  - Brachialis (flexion)

- Hip joint
  - Gluteus maximus (extension and external rotation)
  - Iliopsoas (flexion and external rotation)
  - Semitendinosus (extension) ⎤ Hamstrings
  - Semimembranosus (extension) ⎦
  - Rectus femoris (flexion)
  - Biceps femoris (extension) - Hamstrings
  - Adductor longus (adduction and external rotation)
- Knee joint
  - Rectus femoris (extension [hip extended]) QUADS
  - Vastus lateralis, intermedius, and medialis (extension [hip flexed])
  - Biceps femoris (flexion and external rotation) ⎤
  - Semimembranosus (flexion and internal rotation) ⎬ HAMSTRINGS
  - Semitendinosus (flexion and internal rotation) ⎦
- Ankle joint
  - Tibialis anterior (dorsiflexion at ankle, inversion at foot)
  - Tibialis posterior (plantar flexion at ankle, inversion of foot)
  - Gastrocnemius (plantar flexion at ankle)
  - Soleus (plantar flexion at ankle)
  - Peroneus longus and brevis (plantar flexion at ankle, eversion at foot)

Depending on the particular movement, each muscle at the involved joint will act as *initiates* either the primary mover or a stabilizer. You need to understand the full mechanics of a joint so that you can effectively analyze participants' movements and pinpoint a specific strong or weak muscle.

Hip flexors.
Iliacus psoas

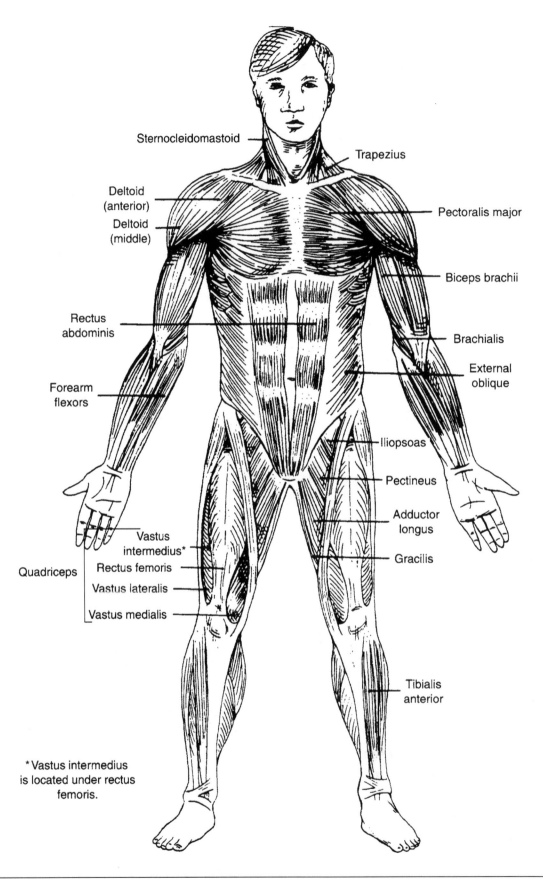

Sternocleidomastoid

Trapezius

Deltoid
(anterior)

Pectoralis major

Deltoid
(middle)

Biceps brachii

Rectus
abdominis

Brachialis

External
oblique

Forearm
flexors

Iliopsoas

Pectineus

Adductor
longus

Vastus
intermedius*

Gracilis

Quadriceps

Rectus femoris

Vastus lateralis

Vastus medialis

Tibialis
anterior

*Vastus intermedius
is located under rectus
femoris.

Figure 5.2 Muscles of the human body—anterior view.

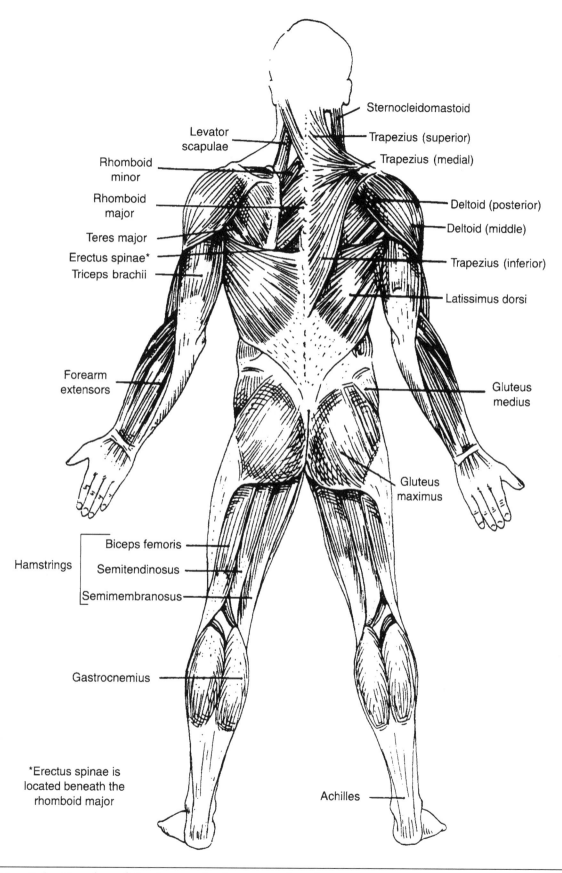

Sternocleidomastoid

Levator
scapulae

Trapezius (superior)

Rhomboid
minor

Trapezius (medial)

Rhomboid
major

Deltoid (posterior)

Teres major

Deltoid (middle)

Erectus spinae*

Trapezius (inferior)

Triceps brachii

Latissimus dorsi

Forearm
extensors

Gluteus
medius

Gluteus
maximus

Hamstrings

Biceps femoris

Semitendinosus

Semimembranosus

Gastrocnemius

*Erectus spinae is
located beneath the
rhomboid major

Achilles

Figure 5.3   Muscles of the human body—posterior view.

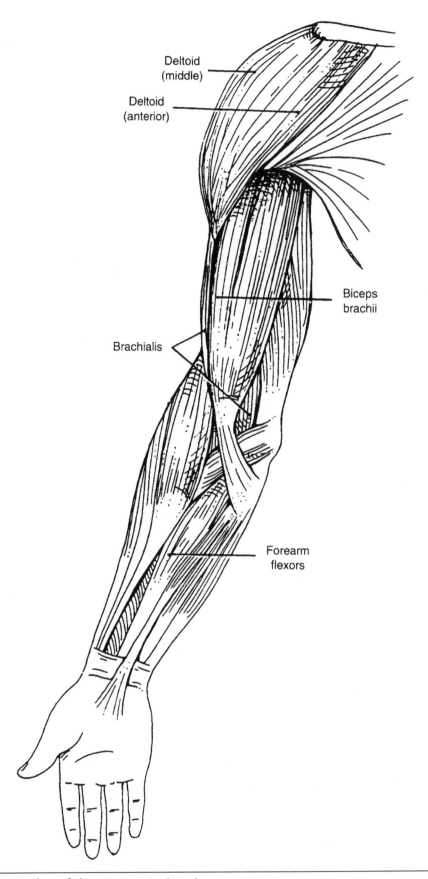

Deltoid
(middle)

Deltoid
(anterior)

Biceps
brachii

Brachialis

Forearm
flexors

Figure 5.4 Muscles of the arm—anterior view.

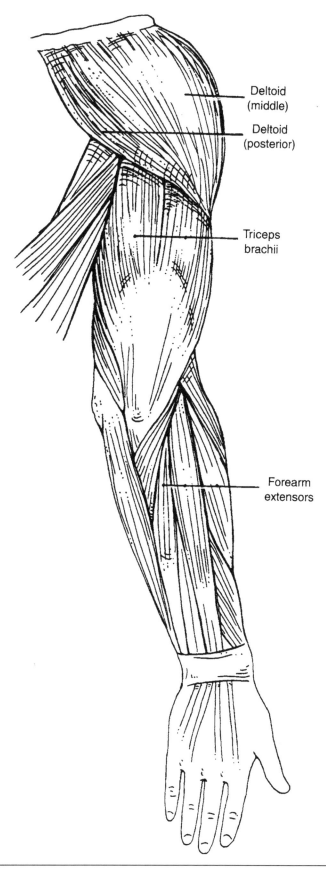

Deltoid
(middle)

Deltoid
(posterior)

Triceps
brachii

Forearm
extensors

Figure 5.5   Muscles of the arm—posterior view.

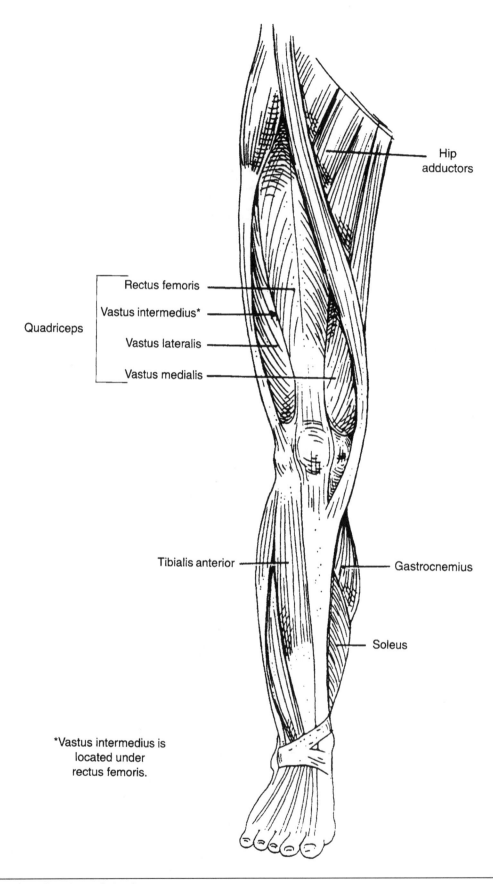

Quadriceps
  Rectus femoris
  Vastus intermedius*
  Vastus lateralis
  Vastus medialis

Hip adductors

Tibialis anterior

Gastrocnemius

Soleus

*Vastus intermedius is located under rectus femoris.

Figure 5.6 Muscles of the leg—anterior view.

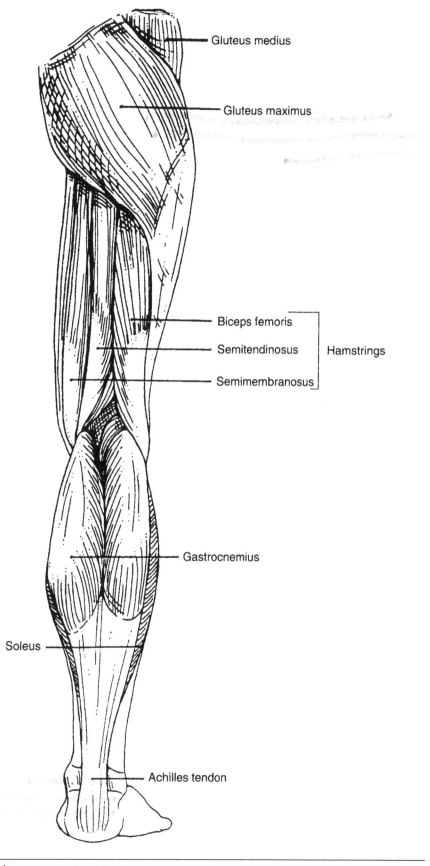

Gluteus medius

Gluteus maximus

Biceps femoris
Semitendinosus   Hamstrings
Semimembranosus

Gastrocnemius

Soleus

Achilles tendon

Figure 5.7 Muscles of the leg—posterior view.

The Spine

The spine is the center of all movement of the human body and the structural foundation of bones that support the body's muscles and soft tissue. The spine is composed of 33 bones called vertebrae: 7 cervical, 12 thoracic, 5 lumbar, 5 sacral, and 4 coccyx (see figure 5.8). The 7 cervical vertebrae are responsible for holding the head up on the frame and have the greatest amount of mobility in the spinal column. The 12 thoracic vertebrae begin the formation of the rib cage (see figures 5.9 and 5.10). The first 7 of these have very little mobility because ribs are attached to them in back and the sternum in front. Thoracic vertebrae numbers 8 through 10 have a bit more mobility because they are attached to the false ribs, and numbers 11 and 12 have the greatest mobility because they are attached to the floating ribs, which have no anterior attachment. The 5 lumbar vertebrae are much larger and stronger than the rest of the vertebrae and allow for a great amount of movement. In addition, they bear the greatest amount of force from gravity and from the fact that they support much of the body weight. Below the lumbar vertebrae is the sacrum, which is 5 vertebrae fused together and limited in movement. Finally, at the base of the

(handwritten margin notes: cervical, thoracic, lumbar)

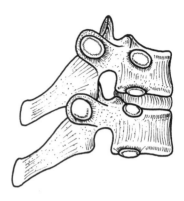

Figure 5.9 Two typical thoracic vertebrae.
Reprinted, by permission, from J. Watkins, 1999, *Structure and function of the musculoskeletal system.* (Champaign, IL: Human Kinetics), 65.

spine is the coccyx, or tailbone, which is 4 small vertebrae fused together. Excluding the sacrum and coccyx, there is a soft disk between each vertebra that cushions impact and movement between the vertebrae.

The spinal column has three natural curvatures that provide both strength and flexibility. Starting at the top, there is a lordodic, or forward, curve in the cervical region; a kyphotic, or backward, curve in the thoracic region; and another lordodic curve in the lumbar region. A spine in proper alignment will maintain the integrity of these curves with equal amounts of force placed on the disks. Postural misalignments and structural deviations such as the three syndromes described earlier will place too much pressure on one side or the other of one or more disks, causing pressure on a nerve and producing pain (see figure 5.11). Any deviation in spinal alignment will have detrimental effects on other parts of the body, because the body will make adjustments to accommodate the deviation, compounding the misalignment.

The spine is unique in that it is one of the few structures of the body that both provides stability and is highly mobile. In Pilates mat exercise, participants will learn to stabilize the spine as well as keep it in proper alignment throughout movement. Unfortunately, with inactivity the muscles that support and move the spine become weak and inflexible, and mobility becomes limited. This is what Joseph

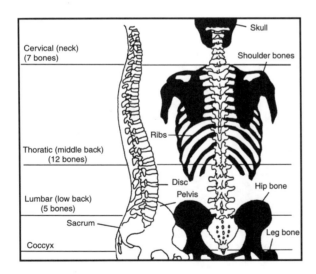

Figure 5.8 Side and back views of spine.
Reprinted, by permission, from YMCA of the USA, 2001, *YMCA healthy back program instructor's guide.* (Champaign, IL: Human Kinetics), 10.

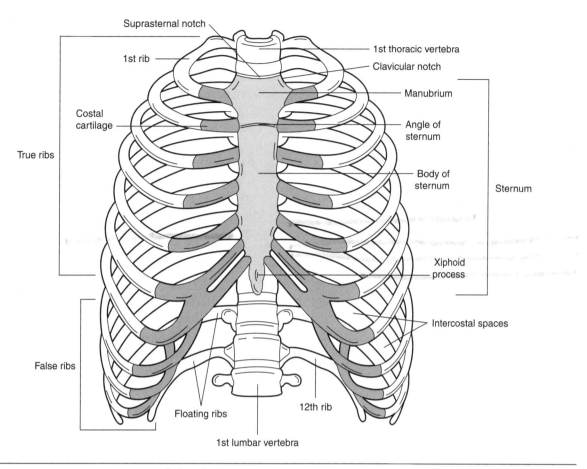

Figure 5.10 Anterior view of the thorax.

Reprinted, by permission, from R.S. Behnke, 2001, *Kinetic anatomy.* (Champaign, IL: Human Kinetics), 158.

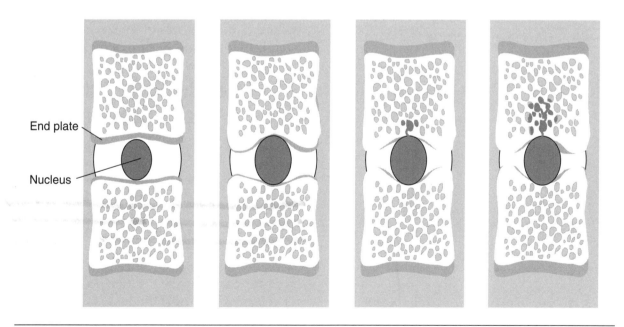

Figure 5.11 Compression of a vertebral disk.

Reprinted, by permission, from S. McGill, 2002, *Low back disorders: evidence-based prevention and rehabilitation.* (Champaign, IL: Human Kinetics), 50.

Pilates was referring to when he spoke about age in relation to spinal flexibility. He stated, "If your spine is inflexibly stiff at 30, you are old; if it is completely flexible at 60, you are young" (Pilates and Miller 1998, p. 16). Learning movement through the spine is imperative for overall health and functionality of the body (see figure 5.12). The spine's condition has a major impact on a person's health and vitality.

Pilates teaches a technique called *rolling through the spine*, or articulating the spine, which means to mindfully place one vertebra at a time on the floor when going from a sitting position to lying flat on the back and to reverse that as you bring the body back up. Beginning participants are usually so unaware of the spine and its mobility that this type of movement is quite difficult initially. You will need to help participants gain awareness and focus when learning this movement and others like it, by using specific verbal cues such as "Roll up one vertebra at a time" and "Roll down one vertebra at a time." With practice, participants will be able to gradually increase their ROM, gaining precision of movement.

Rolling through Spine

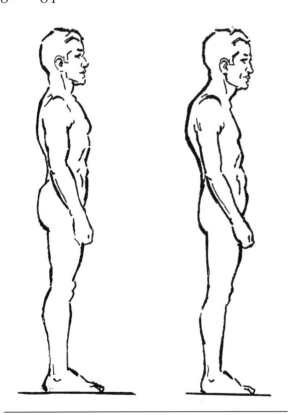

Figure 5.12 Changes in posture as a result of inactivity.

Many exercise practitioners often refer to a *neutral spine* as a desirable alignment position. A true neutral spine is when it is in its most natural position, with normal curvatures in the cervical, thoracic, and lumbar areas. In this position, the vertebrae align evenly on each disk so that there is no undue pressure or discomfort. Maintaining a neutral spine is fairly easy to accomplish when standing, but more challenging when the body is in other positions. To understand how to meet this challenge, consider the following example of how to achieve a neutral spine in a back-lying position: Place the base of the hands on top of the hip bones with fingertips pointing down at the pelvis. Use the hands to level out the hip bones and the pelvis, and the natural lordodic curvature of the lumbar area should result. The accompanying contraction of the abdomen will keep the pelvis in proper position.

The spinal column can sustain a great deal of force and allow for quite a range of mobility because the vertebrae and disks are designed to withstand a normal amount of impact and movement that occur during daily activity. You should teach participants to be conscious of proper posture and positioning not only during Pilates classes but also during their other workouts and daily life activities as well. By repeating correct technique, participants will minimize chances of injury and improve overall strength and flexibility over time.

The Body's Core Musculature

If the spinal column is considered the structural foundation of the body, the core musculature must be considered its powerhouse. The core involves the muscles of the trunk—the abdomen, pelvis, and back, which function to both move and stabilize the spine. With proper engagement of the core muscles, the spine becomes fully protected and stable. This stability creates the desirable postural position where the chest is lifted, the shoulders are pulled back and down, and the abdominal muscles are held in. If there is improper alignment anywhere along the spine, a participant can be taught to use specific and focused contraction of core musculature to bring it back into place for proper posture. Once the participant achieves and maintains strength and flexibility of the core musculature, the spine will be able to resume its proper, natural alignment and the torso will appear more erect.

The stronger the core muscles are, the more resilient the body becomes to injuries and misalignments. Using a push-up exercise as an example, the important supporting role of the core musculature can be seen in maintaining proper body alignment and form. If the participant's core is weak, the back will not be able to support itself during this movement, and it will sag toward the floor (see figure 5.13a). This lack of support will result in undue stress on the lower spine, as well as on the shoulders and neck region, and the participant will perform the exercise in a weak, inefficient manner. On the other hand, if the core is strong, the participant will hold the torso in a straight position, evenly distribute weight on the joints, and perform the exercise without undue musculoskeletal stress (see figure 5.13b).

Pilates mat exercise focuses on the postural placement and engagement of the core muscles.

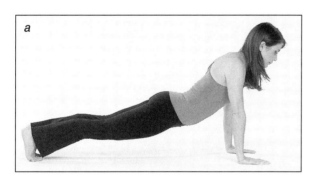

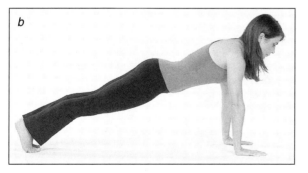

Figure 5.13 (a) Incorrect push-up form because core muscles are not engaged. (b) Correct push-up form with core engagement.

In a standing position, correct postural alignment includes lowering the shoulders and opening the chest by pulling the shoulders back. It also emphasizes contracting the abdomen and pulling the rib cage in and down toward the pelvis instead of being extended outward. This action helps the pelvis be level to allow for proper lumbar region curvature and a neutral spine. You will teach participants to maintain this alignment even while they expand the breath by breathing from the lungs, not the lower portion of the abdomen. In Pilates exercise, breathing should never compromise the integrity of the core muscles: The rib cage should remain contracted and the breath should expand by contraction of the diaphragm. In addition, maintaining a contraction in the lower portion of the abdomen will enable the diaphragm to work in its appropriate manner.

The Abdomen

The abdominal muscles play a key role in core strength and mobility (see figure 5.14). Three muscles constitute the abdominal area:

1. Rectus abdominis
2. Internal and external obliques
3. Transverse abdominis (see figure 5.15)

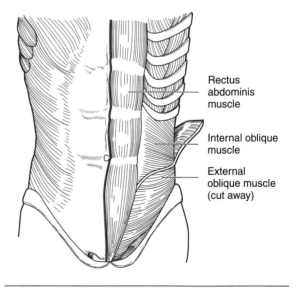

Rectus abdominis muscle

Internal oblique muscle

External oblique muscle (cut away)

Figure 5.14 Muscles of the abdominal wall.

Reprinted, by permission, from C.M. Norris, 2000, *Back stability*. (Champaign, IL: Human Kinetics), 57.

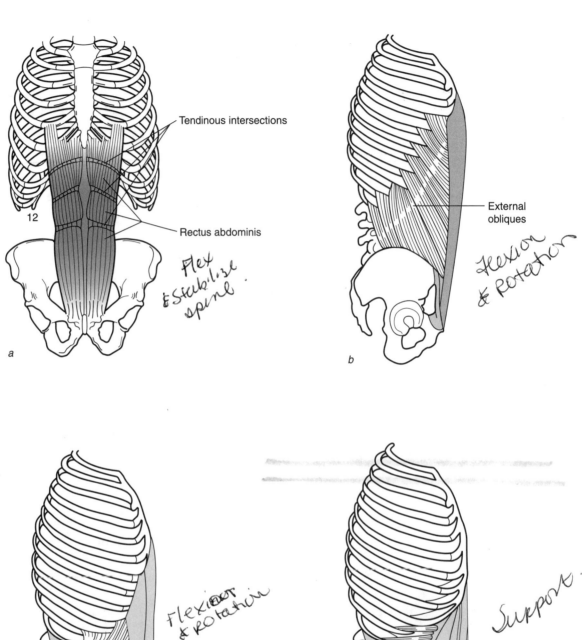

Tendinous intersections

Rectus abdominis

Flex & Stabilize spine.

12

a

External obliques

Flexion & Rotation

b

Internal obliques

Flexion EXT & Rotation

c

Transversus abdominis

Support.

d

Figure 5.15 *(a)* The linea alba and rectus abdominis. *(b)* The external obliques. *(c)* The internal obliques. *(d)* The transversus abdominis.

Reprinted, by permission, from R.S. Behnke, 2001, *Kinetic anatomy.* (Champaign, IL: Human Kinetics), 143.

Developing control of the abdominal muscles is one of the first concepts and techniques for Pilates participants to grasp. The first step in this process is to learn the anatomical orientation of the abdomen. The *rectus abdominis* runs from the rib cage to the pelvis and is designed to flex as well as stabilize the spine. The *internal and external obliques* run alongside the rectus abdominis on the sides of the trunk and together perform spinal flexion and rotation. The *transverse abdominis* is the deepest of the group, and it encircles the abdominal cavity. Together these muscles provide a base of support for the area between the rib cage and the pelvis and are an integral part of the powerhouse to which Joseph Pilates referred. If these muscles lose conditioning from either lack of exercise or incorrect posture, they become too weak to adequately support the spine. This lack of support creates an exaggerated lumbar lordosis and causes uneven pressure on the disks, increasing the potential for back pain and injury. The muscles of the abdominal area must be conditioned through regular exercise to maintain strength and flexibility. It is important to exercise all three abdominal muscles in order to promote balance and stability of the area. While exercise participants usually address the rectus abdominis and oblique muscles, they often ignore the transverse abdominis. Beginning Pilates participants will notice that it takes some time and work for the transverse abdominis to catch up in strength to the rest of the group. When it does, they will experience significantly improved alignment of the pelvis and stability of the spine.

Participants will have to learn how to contract the abdominal muscles without using a *sucking in* movement, which interferes with breathing and the stabilization of the spine. When participants contract the abdomen appropriately, they maintain the natural curvatures of the spine. These natural curvatures are the correct position for the spine and should remain present throughout movement.

The Pelvis

The pelvis, located approximately in the middle of the body, transfers forces from the upper body to the lower body through its union with the large thigh bone, the femur. It also helps absorb the forces that are generated by the lower body and lessens them as they move up the spine.

Both the sacral portion of the spine and the two femur bones are anchored to the pelvis, making it important to maintain proper pelvic positioning in order to maintain the integrity of those joints. For proper positioning to occur, the anterior and posterior muscles of the body must work in unison. Any deviation in the relative strength of these muscles will create an imbalance, tilting the pelvis forward or backward, affecting alignment and posture.

After learning to control the movement of the abdominal muscles, Pilates participants will focus on controlling the pelvis. For an example of pelvic muscle control, consider when an exercise instructor tells participants to squeeze the buttocks to help stabilize the core. In reality, there are two separate movements that should occur to accomplish this—first, a tightening of the gluteal muscles and then a motion to tuck them in. Beginners will instinctively perform these movements at the same time, but Pilates participants will learn to differentiate between the two movements and control each one.

On the anterior, or front, side of the body, the abdominal muscles are responsible for pulling the pelvis upward, while the hip flexors pull downward. On the posterior, or back, side of the body, the back muscles pull the pelvis upward, and the hip extensors pull downward. If the muscle group on one side of the body exerts greater force than the other, the pelvis will tilt in that direction, causing misalignment and poor posture. As long as these two teams of muscles have balanced strength and flexibility, they will hold the pelvis in perfect alignment for the rest of the body (see figure 5.16).

Movement Modifications

It is essential that fitness instructors, particularly those teaching Pilates exercise, develop the skills of observing movement and recommending corrective actions. The more you

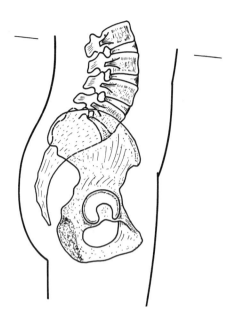

Figure 5.16 Proper pelvis position in standing posture.

Reprinted, by permission, from J. Watkins, 1999, *Structure and function of the musculoskeletal system.* (Champaign, IL: Human Kinetics), 175.

understand about the interrelationships of the muscles and joints of the body, the more effective you will be at analyzing movement, pinpointing areas to address, and creating appropriate modifications. In addition to providing specific movement tips, instructors will need to continually remind participants to focus the

mind on their actions. Training participants to become more focused on the movement of the body will help them understand and master the details of each Pilates exercise. To facilitate this, you must be able to provide specific visual, verbal, and tactile cues that will result in the desired movement. When viewing and analyzing participant movement, remember to always start from the core, because poor or incorrect technique often can be traced to that area. Once the core is stable and functioning correctly, continue the analysis outward to the rest of the body. Use the following checklist to make modifications in Pilates mat exercise:

- Review the core and neutral spine for any postural deviations.

- Keep in mind that the longer the lever, the more challenging a movement will be for the participant. For example, movements or positions with legs extended are more challenging than those movements with legs bent in towards the chest.

- During the initial stages of Pilates training, break each movement down to its basic components, gradually adding a level of complexity as participants master each phase.

- Never compromise technique and positioning for speed or number of repetitions.

6

The YMCA Pilates Mat Work Program

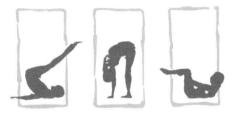

In Joseph Pilates's original publication of his exercises in 1945, he prescribed 34 exercises to be performed regularly for optimal results. In this chapter, we describe in detail the 29 Pilates exercises and variations chosen to be included in the YMCA Pilates program. Prior to the specific exercises, we introduce a postural identification process to help teach participants how to assume a desirable starting position for exercising. After that, we cover a warm-up sequence that includes breathing, spinal positioning, shoulder retraction, and an abdominal crunch. The third section of the chapter includes all the exercise descriptions, beginning with The Hundred on page 42. The final section is information about combining the exercises together in various class formats.

It should be noted that although we describe 29 exercises and 3 different combinations or sequences in this manual, only the first 21 exercises and 2 sequences are taught in the YMCA of the USA Pilates Instructor certification course. Because of the additional time needed to master the more advanced exercises, the course focuses on the beginning and intermediate exercises, which give the instructor a solid base to begin instruction and are sufficient for beginner and intermediate mat exercise classes.

Exercise Overview

The YMCA Pilates mat work program consists of a total of 29 exercises that use the entire body, presented in three different sequences for learning progression and flow. Each exercise is as valuable as the next, and each exercise must be mastered before moving on to the next. Participants will find that each exercise in Pilates actually comprises several smaller movements that together make the complete exercise. Successful practice of Pilates exercise occurs when participants can understand, feel, and emphasize each of those small movements to ensure the success of the entire movement. Following is a list of the warm-up sequence and all the mat exercises included in the YMCA Pilates Program:

- The Warm-up sequence
  - Deep abdominal breathing
  - Neutral spine and spinal imprinting
  - Shoulder retraction
  - Abdominal crunch
- Mat exercises
  1. The Hundred
  2. Assisted Roll-Up

3. Roll-Up
4. Roll-Over
5. Single-Leg Circle
6. Rolling
7. Single-Leg Stretch
8. Double-Leg Stretch
9. Scissors
10. Spine Stretch
11. Leg Lowers
12. Rocking
13. Corkscrew
14. Saw
15. Swan
16. Single-Leg Kick
17. Double-Leg Kick
18. Bicycle Twist
19. The Bridge
20. Side-Leg Kick Series
21. Seal
22. Neck Pull*
23. Spine Twist*
24. Jackknife*
25. Teaser Prep*
26. Hip Circles*
27. Swimming*
28. Leg-Pull Front*
29. Push-Up*

* More advanced exercises not included in the YMCA Pilates Instructor certification course.

Note that the exercises are listed in this order for reference only. See the suggested class sequences of exercises at the end of this chapter on pages 80 to 84.

As you teach the Pilates mat exercises in a class, you may focus on and repeat a movement many times to help participants master it before progressing to the next. During the learning stages, you may repeat movements five to eight times. Once movements are mastered, the repe-

titions will decrease to two to three times. In the early stages of teaching an exercise, the key is to use the repetitions as a learning tool without creating fatigue that may distract the mind and cause a loss of focus on the body's movements. You may find that participants need to work on specific exercises and techniques each time the class meets. One of the benefits of Pilates exercise is that you may employ a great deal of flexibility in structuring each class, depending on individual needs. Unlike traditional exercise, advancement in Pilates exercise is not necessarily doing more exercise, but mastering each exercise. Accomplishing this mastery may take much repetition over extended periods of time. Once participants have mastered all of the individual movements, the flow from movement to movement will begin to be more efficient, the amount of repetitions needed will decrease, and participants will begin to develop a unity of mind and body in movement.

The first sequence to learn is Pilates Mat Work 1, composed of 11 beginning movements. After mastering this first level of movements, participants will move on to Pilates Mat Work 2, which consists of 13 exercises—10 new movements and 3 repeated from Mat Work 1. Participants should now have mastered the basic principles of movement, making progression faster than in Mat Work 1. Again, you may repeat the new exercises more than usual until participants have accomplished the mind–body connection, remembering that the perfection of the movement is more important than speed and repetitions. Once mastered, exercises from Mat Work 1 and 2 can be combined to create an intermediate-level class. Pilates Mat Work 3 consists of 18 exercises, 8 new, more advanced movements, and 10 repeated from the prior sequences. Once these are mastered, exercises from Mat Work 1, 2, and 3 can be combined for an advanced-level class.

For a number of the exercises in all three levels, you have the option to use various props to enhance the movement. Keep in mind that you should use props only if participants have mastered the initial movement.

Postural Identification

Before starting the warm-up you should help participants check their basic body position that they should be in for Pilates exercise. Following is a description of the desired position to begin exercising:

1. **Initial positioning:** Lie down on your back with the knees bent, feet flat on the mat (hip-width apart), and the arms resting on the mat by the sides.
2. Lengthen the neck with the chin back toward the spine and slightly down. Think of the space between the chin and the chest as being equivalent to the size of an egg.
3. Keep the shoulders back and down. *Relax shoulders down your back*
4. ~~Elevate the chest.~~ *No*
5. Hold the rib cage in and down.
6. Contract the abdominal muscles.
7. Neutralize the spine.

The movements in the following warm-up sequence are designed for you to begin teaching participants proper alignment, breathing, awareness, and some basic movement patterns. With practice, you will begin to recognize faulty movement patterns during the warm-up movements. Use this information to begin teaching participants where their bodies are in space, creating the kinesthetic awareness that will maximize form and technique in the exercises that follow.

The Warm-Up

For the Pilates mat work series, the warm-up is an opportunity for participants to prepare for purposeful movement by becoming more aware of the body's positioning and its movements, and their breathing. The warm-up sequence includes deep abdominal breathing, spinal positioning and imprinting, shoulder retraction, and abdominal crunch.

⓵ *Deep Abdominal Breathing*

Keep in mind that the average person is unaware of a proper breathing technique to use during exercise. By teaching deep abdominal breathing, you can show participants how to properly breathe and create an optimal flow of breath with movement.

1. **Initial positioning:** Lie down on your back with the knees bent and the feet flat on the mat, hip-width apart, and arms resting on the mat by the sides.

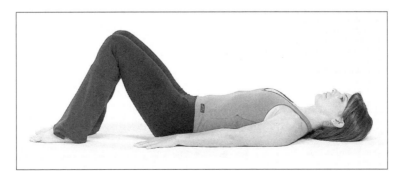

2. **First phase of movement:** Pull the shoulders down and back into the mat and contract the abdominal muscles with focus on the lower section of the muscles. Place both hands on the rib cage and breathe in through the nose and out through the mouth, expanding the rib cage on the inhalation, and contracting when you breathe out through the mouth. Maintain the contraction in the lower section of the abdominal muscles throughout the breath.

3. **Second phase of movement:** Minimize the movement in the rib cage while maintaining the abdominal contraction. Allow the diaphragm and lungs to work as one with each breath. During the exhalation, allow the rib cage to contract further; this will assist in the complete removal of air from the lungs.

②*Neutral Spine and Spinal Imprinting*

This procedure will help participants begin to discover body awareness and positioning. First, you will teach them how to position the body for a neutral spine, and then they will move on to spinal imprinting while maintaining this position.

1. **Initial positioning:** Lie down on your back with the knees bent and the feet flat on the mat, hip-width apart.

2. **First phase of movement:** Place the palm of the hand on the outer edges of the pelvis with the fingertips on the pubic bone, using the hands to tilt the pelvis so that the palms of the hands and the fingertips are level and parallel to the floor.

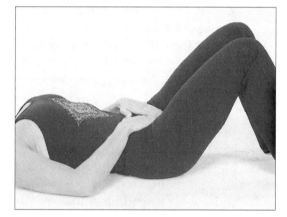

3. **Second phase of movement:** If needed, keep the hands on the pelvis to maintain an awareness of the pelvis and rib cage. Otherwise, let the hands rest on the floor. Inhale and bring one knee into the chest while extending the leg up toward the ceiling. Exhale and lower the straight leg down toward the floor, dragging the foot back to the starting position. Repeat the sequence on the other side. (Repeat movements on both sides two to three times). Spinal imprinting takes place by allowing the spine to release into the mat without moving the pelvis from the neutral position during the entire movement.

4. **Movement considerations:**
   * If participants bring the knee too far into the chest, the pelvis will shift.
   * The breath should be deep with little to no movement in the rib cage.
   * Be aware that when the leg is extended up, the pelvis may shift, particularly if participants try to get the leg up to 90 degrees. Remind them that the degree of extension can be modified so that the pelvis does not change positioning because this is a prime focus of this movement.
   * When lowering the leg, the pelvis will shift if the abdominal muscles are weak. Teach participants to bend the knee right at the point before the pelvis shifts in order to maintain the desired pelvic positioning.

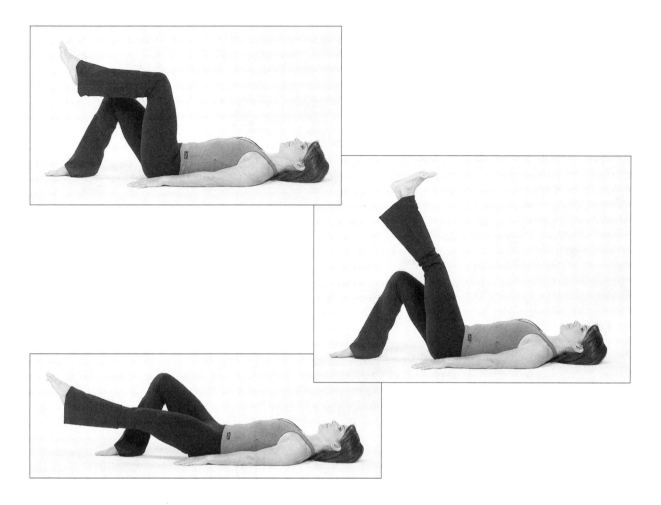

③ *Shoulder Retraction*

In many individuals, shoulders are elevated and brought forward because of weak or tight muscles as well as poor postural habits. Retraction teaches participants how to move the scapulae and retrain the rhomboids to maintain proper posture and shoulder positioning throughout exercise as well as daily movements.

1. **Initial positioning:** Lie down on your back with the knees bent and the feet flat on the mat, hip-width apart. Maintain a neutral spine and allow only minimal movement in the rib cage.

2. **First phase of movement:** Reach straight up toward the ceiling with both arms. With the palms facing each other, squeeze the shoulder blades together during the inhalation phase of breathing and allow them to separate on the exhalation.

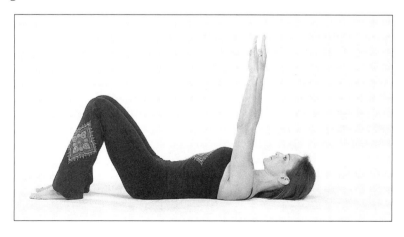

3. **Second phase of movement:** Continue moving the arms overhead, lowering them onto the mat above the head. While maintaining the neutral spine and the rib cage placement, squeeze and retract the shoulder blades down toward the hips.

Inhale during this motion as you bring the arms up toward the ceiling above the shoulders at the same time. Next, exhale and return the arms to the initial position on the mat. Repeat the movement 3 times.

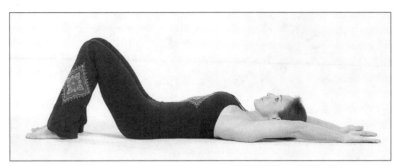

4. **Movement considerations:**

   - The goal of the initial phase of movement is to become aware of the movement of the scapulae without losing the integrity of the spine and the torso. Remind participants to keep their shoulders down and back.

   - During the second phase, the rib cage will naturally tend to open once the arms are above the head. This is the point where the participants need to stay focused to maintain the integrity in the torso. This will become a vivid example of the importance of the mind–body connection.

   - The focus of the second phase is not on the arm movement. The real objective is to move the scapulae down and together, which in turn will assist in moving the arms. It is important that participants understand this principle and methodology because it will assist them in learning all the moves to follow.

5. **Props:** For a variation requiring a bit more strength and balance, this same movement can be done with a stability ball placed under the head and shoulders. The movement is the same as described previously, except that the shoulder blades move into the ball rather than into the mat.

Abdominal Crunch

Developing control of the abdominal muscles is one of the basic principles of Pilates exercise. This control must be learned early in Pilates training, because it is essential for mastering this exercise program. Maintaining core stability by correctly engaging the abdominal muscles will be the basis for many of the movements to follow. As seen in the previous exercise, each movement will have one or more underlying components that play a role in creating it. Once participants can learn to focus and control each of these components, they will begin to experience noticeable benefits.

1. **Initial positioning:** Lie down on your back with the knees bent and the feet flat on the mat, hip-width apart, and with the arms raised just up off of the mat, by the sides. Maintain a neutral spine and allow only minimal movement in the rib cage.

2. **Movement components:** Inhale and push the shoulders back and down toward the hips, which will allow the neck to lengthen. Exhale and contract the rib cage in toward the pelvis as you lift the upper body off the mat as one unit. Inhale and lower back down. Repeat the movement three times.

3. **Movement considerations:**
   - Once the neck is lengthened, its position should not change, even during the contraction of the rib cage.
   - As the rib cage contracts down toward the pelvis, the bend will feel as though it occurs at the navel. Teach this position with the verbal cue, "It is as if you are bending in two at the belly button."
   - If participants experience neck discomfort, try to have them realign the neck positioning. If discomfort continues, have them place the hands behind the head without changing the positioning of the rest of the body.

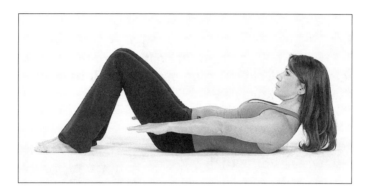

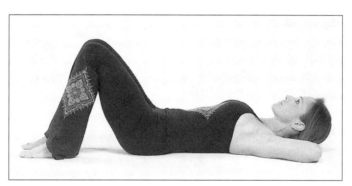

4. **Props:** For a variation requiring a bit more strength and balance, this same movement can be done with a stability ball placed under the lower back. The movement is the same as described previously with an added emphasis on neck alignment.

The Exercises

Following are detailed descriptions of the 29 Pilates mat exercises in the YMCA program, each with the exercise goal, initial position, movement components and breathing, verbal cueing suggestions, modifications and use of props, and teaching tips.

1. THE HUNDRED

Goals

Challenge the abdominals and thoroughly warm up the body by engaging all the areas of the body that will be working during the mat routine.

Initial Positioning

Lie down on your back with the arms by the sides of the body and the knees bent with the feet flat on the mat.

Movement Components and Breathing

Exhale and contract the rib cage down to the pelvis while lifting the scapula off the floor with the palms facing down, similar to a crunch movement. Inhale and return to the beginning position. Repeat the movement 3 times.

With the upper body held in the crunch position, inhale and lift the feet off of the floor, keeping the knees bent and holding the lower legs parallel to the floor. From this position, pump the arms toward the mat three times with the palms down as you exhale, then pump the arms with the palms up three times as you inhale. (Note: As participants' lung capacity and ability to use the breath correctly increases, the arm may pump as many as five times with each inhalation and exhalation). Progress to pumping the arms a total of 100 times.

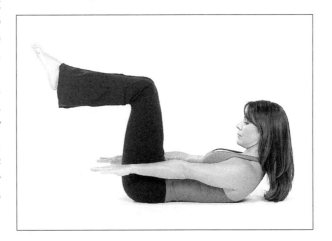

Verbal Cueing Suggestions

- "Pull the shoulders back and down."
- "Keep a neutral spine."
- "Contract the abdominal muscles and rib cage."

Modifications

- Novice: Instead of lifting the feet off of the floor, keep both feet flat on the floor.
- Advanced: From the crunch position, extend the legs straight up toward the ceiling, maintaining the integrity of the core muscles. A more difficult option still is to lower the straight legs closer toward the floor, holding them just off the floor.

Teaching Tips

Be sure to continually cue your participants so that they maintain their awareness of all the components of the movement. If participants experience neck pain, first realign them to make sure they have the correct crunch position. If it continues, have them rest the head on the mat with a rolled-up towel under the neck for support.

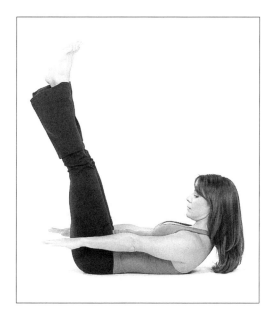
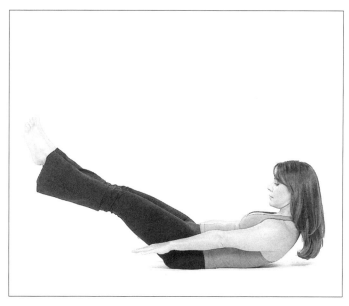

Props

- Flat resistance band: Place the band around the soles of the feet and extend the legs to the ceiling. Hold the ends firmly with the hands, and maintain this static stretch position.
- Magic Circle: Place the Magic Circle between the ankles and engage the muscles of the inner thighs to hold it in place.

2. ASSISTED ROLL-UP

Goal

Introduce the concept of engaging and integrating the core muscles while lifting or peeling the spine off the mat one vertebra at a time and imprinting it on the way back down.

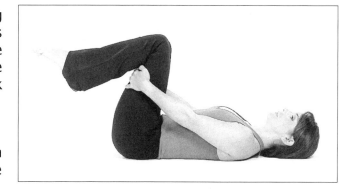

Initial Positioning

Lie down on your back with the knees pulled in toward the chest.

Movement Components and Breathing

Inhale and place the hands behind the knees. Exhale, contract the abdominal muscles, move the rib cage down toward the pelvis, and begin to roll up one vertebra at a time. During the roll-up, also press the legs against the hands to assist the body as it comes to a seated position with the legs flat on the mat. From here, reach forward with the hands toward the feet. Inhale, exhale and roll back down, reversing the initial movement. Repeat the movement three to five times.

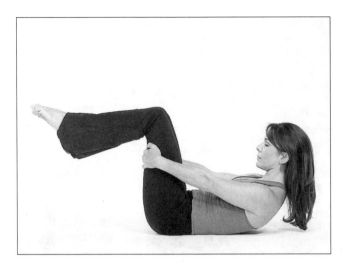
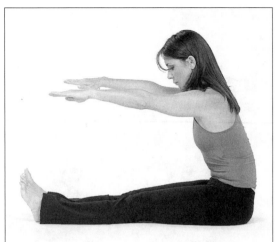

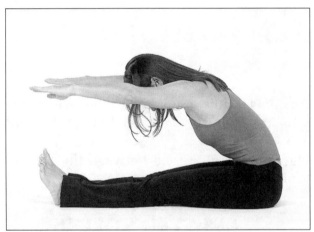

Verbal Cueing Suggestions

- "Lift with the abdominal muscles and back muscles, using the hands to help, if needed."
- "Roll down one vertebra at a time."

Modifications

Novice: If this movement is difficult, have the participants limit their movement range of motion.

Teaching Tips

Most participants will pull with the hands against the back of the legs more than needed, often because doing so requires less concentration and effort. Keep participants focused on the components of the movement. Being able to roll up without assistance is a positive indication of participants' improvements in strength.

Props

Flat resistance band: Place the band around the soles of the feet and hold the ends with both hands. Use the tension in the band to assist with the movement in both directions.

3. THE ROLL-UP

Goal

Engage the abdominal muscles to both roll the body off the floor in a peeling motion without using momentum in the lifting and to maintain stabilization in the lower body.

Initial Positioning

Lie down on your back with arms extended over the head and the legs extended straight out on the mat with the feet neutral.

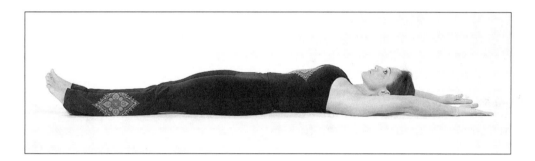

Movement Components and Breathing

As you exhale, contract the rib cage toward the pelvis and begin to lift the upper body, peeling up one vertebra at a time. Keep the arms extended, legs active, and abdominals contracted as you continue rolling up off the mat. As the abdominal muscles become fully contracted, reach the arms toward the legs, keep the shoulders depressed, and extend the legs. Begin to inhale and reverse the movements back down to the starting position. Repeat the movement five to eight times.

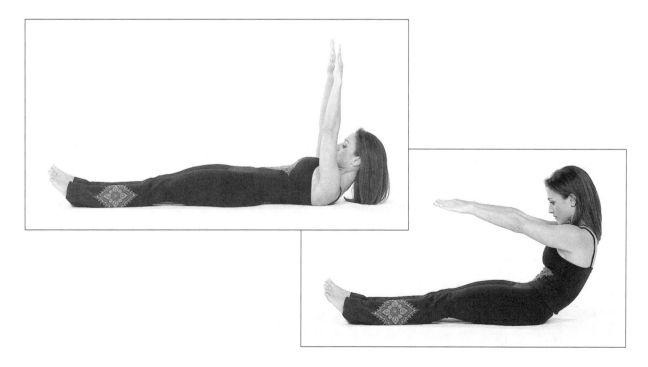

Verbal Cueing Suggestions

- "Pull the shoulders back and down."
- "Keep a neutral spine."
- "Lift with the abdominal muscles and rib cage." (You should see a slight contraction in the inner thighs and hamstrings, which anchor the abdominal muscles.)

Modifications

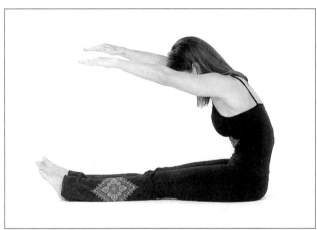

- Novice: If unable to perform the Roll-Up, perform the Assisted Roll-Up (on pages 43–44) instead until you have developed more strength. The next progression is to perform the roll-up with bent knees instead of straight legs.
- Advanced: Keep the arms extended overhead throughout the movement instead of reaching for the legs.

Teaching Tips

If the neck alignment is compromised, the muscles in that area will tighten and become uncomfortable. If this happens, have participants place one or both hands behind the head, keeping the torso in proper alignment.

Props

Magic Circle: Place the Magic Circle between the hands and keep it in place by slightly pressing inward with the hands.

4. THE ROLL-OVER

Goal

Strengthen the core muscles by using them to lift the lower body up over the head.

Initial Positioning

Lie down on your back with the arms resting at the sides of the body and the legs fully extended on the mat.

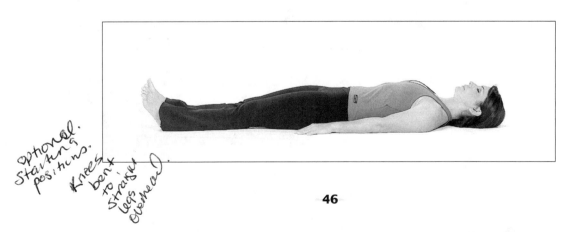

optional.
starting positions.
knees bent to straight legs overhead.

Movement Components and Breathing

Before starting, make sure that the shoulders are pushed down and back into the mat. As you inhale, begin to lift the legs up, keeping them straight, and moving them past vertical to an overhead position where they are parallel to the mat. Exhale, separate the legs, press down with the arms, and allow the body to roll back to the starting position. Repeat the movement five to eight times.

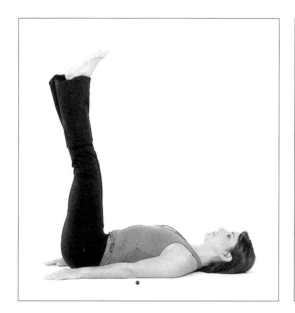 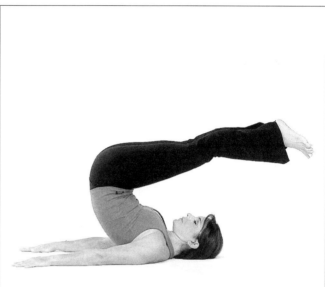

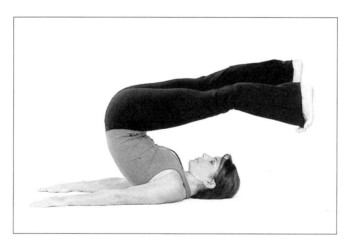

Verbal Cueing Suggestions

- "Maintaining shoulder blade retraction, push down a bit with the arms into the mat to assist the abdominal muscles."
- "Contract the abdominal muscles and rib cage."
- "Keep the legs parallel to the floor." (This will minimize pressure on the neck.)
- "Keep the shoulders back and down."

Modifications

- Novice: Instead of lifting the legs straight, start by bending the knees and lifting them into the chest. From there, extend them up straight to 90 degrees, and proceed from that point. Also, keep the legs together throughout the movement.
- Advanced: Bring the legs all the way over the head, eventually touching the mat on the final phase of the movement.

Teaching Tips

Beginning participants may lack the abdominal muscle strength required to perform this exercise correctly, so you may want to teach the novice modification before progressing to the full movement. Be sure to remind participants to be conscious of engaging the muscles of the body, to do the work in a controlled manner, and not to allow momentum to take over.

Props

Stability ball: Place a stability ball between the feet, and lift the legs up to a 90-degree angle to the floor. Hold the ball in place with the feet and lower the legs overhead toward the floor.

5. SINGLE-LEG CIRCLE

Goal

Increase hip and core stability and inner thigh strength.

Initial Positioning

Lie down on your back with the legs extended straight out, resting on the mat.

Movement Components and Breathing

Keeping one leg extended on the mat, raise the other one straight up, pointing to the ceiling. Inhale and start making a small circle with the straight leg crossing the midline of the body, then exhale and swing the leg out, and circle it back to the starting position. Keep the hips engaged to maintain a neutral spine during the movement. Start with small circles, and then gradually make the circles larger, always maintaining core stability. Repeat the circling motion three to five times. Then lower the leg to the starting position, and repeat the movement with the other leg three to five times.

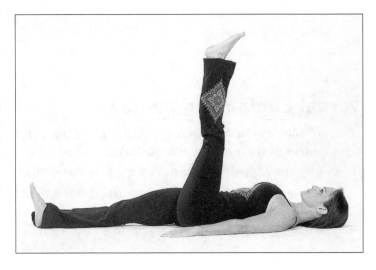

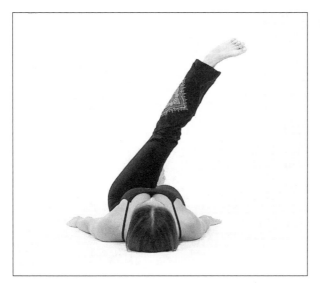
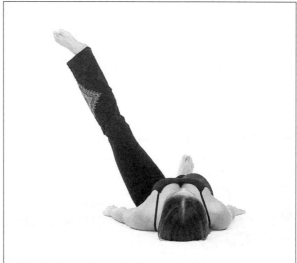

Verbal Cueing Suggestions

- "Keep the abdominal muscles, rib cage, and hips in place as you circle the leg."
- "Keep the neck long, with a neutral spine."
- "Let the hands stay loose."
- "Keep the shoulders down."
- "Increase the size of the circle as long as you can keep the abdominals, rib cage, and hips in place."

Modifications

- Novice: Place the hands on the pelvis to help maintain neutral hips. Bend the leg that is resting on the mat at the knee so that the foot is flat on the floor. *Modified*
- Advanced: Increase the size of the circle so that the leg crosses over the body and is over the floor, without compromising core stability.

Teaching Tips

Remind participants to focus on maintaining proper body positioning as they circle the leg, not just on the movement of the leg.

Props

Flat resistance band: Place the band around the sole of the circling leg's foot, and hold the ends of the band with both hands. Stretch the band slightly to add resistance to the circular movement while maintaining the pelvis in a stable, relaxed position.

6. ROLLING

Goal

Develop <u>abdominal control and balance</u>.

Initial Positioning

Sit with the knees bent into the chest and the feet off the floor, holding the hands on the front of the ankles. In this position, the body is balanced like a ball, with its weight on the sit bones.

Movement Components and Breathing

Keeping the shoulders pressed down, let the head lower down toward the knees. Inhale, contract the abdominal muscles fully, and allow the body to roll backward onto the shoulder blades. Exhale and roll the body back up to the starting position, again balancing on the sit bones, not letting the feet touch the mat. Repeat the movement three to five times.

Verbal Cueing Suggestions

- "Keep your body in the same position throughout the movement."
- "Contract the abdominal muscles and roll with control."

Modifications

- Novice: Limit the movement's ROM just enough so that the participant can control it and return to the starting position. Another modification is to move the hands behind the knees for better support.
- Advanced: Create a tighter or smaller ball shape with the body, without compromising control or positioning.

Teaching Tips

Beginning participants may roll back too far and go all the way onto the head. They must keep control of the rolling so that the movement only goes to the shoulder blades, not onto the neck or head.

Props

None.

7. SINGLE-LEG STRETCH

Goal

Train the pelvis to maintain stability and a neutral spine while moving and stretching the legs in opposition.

Initial Positioning

Lie down on your back with the legs extended straight out on the mat.

Movement Components and Breathing

Raise one knee into the chest and slowly lift the other leg straight off the floor. Elevate the upper body off the floor by contracting the rib cage down toward the pelvis. Reach forward with the hand on the same side as the bent knee to touch the ankle and reach with the other hand to touch the knee. (This positioning helps to align the hip.) As you exhale, switch legs and corresponding hand positioning. Inhale and switch again. One cycle of breathing equals one repetition; repeat three to five times.

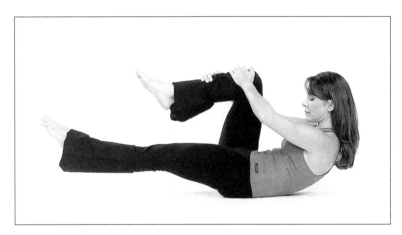

Verbal Cueing Suggestions

- "Keep the abdominal muscles contracted."
- "Keep a neutral spine. Check that the pelvis is not moving from its position."
- "Keep the neck long and in a neutral position." (Even when off the mat, the neck should remain neutral and elongated.)

Modifications

- Novice: Place one hand behind the head. Another modification is to raise the extended leg up higher toward the ceiling, a position from which the participant can better control the movement.
- Advanced: Increase the speed of movement without sacrificing postural integrity.

Teaching Tips

If the movement is performed too fast and without control, participants will often overflex the neck and create undesirable movement in the torso and pelvis.

Props

None.

8. DOUBLE-LEG STRETCH

Goal

Maintain core stabilization during movements of the arms and legs.

Initial Positioning

Lie down on your back with both knees bent up toward the chest, and the lower legs parallel to the floor with feet off the floor. Lift the upper body by contracting the rib cage toward the pelvis and raise arms off the mat, keeping them parallel to the floor.

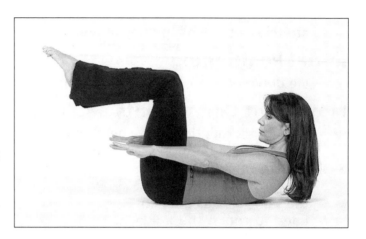

Movement Components and Breathing

Inhale and extend the legs and arms straight up so they are perpendicular to the floor, pointing toward the ceiling. From this position, exhale and simultaneously reach back over the head with the arms and move the legs away from center, down towards the floor, to about a 45-degree angle. Inhale and move the arms from behind the head out to the sides, while maintaining the legs in the same position. Finally, using the abdominal muscles, exhale and draw the knees back in toward the chest, and bring the arms back to the sides. Repeat the movement three to five times.

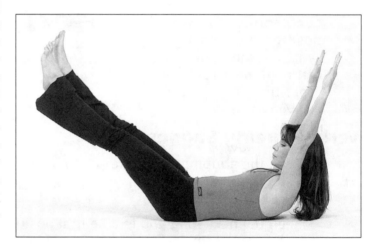

Verbal Cueing Suggestions

- "Contract the abdominal muscles." (This helps maintain the leg and arm extension.)
- "Keep the neck long, in a neutral position."

Modifications

- Novice: Keep the hands behind the head throughout the movement, bringing the elbows together as you inhale, and apart as you exhale. Another modification of hand placement is to hold them on the knees. For the legs, instead of extending them straight out, bend the knees, keeping the lower legs parallel to the floor.
- Advanced: Hold the legs lower to the floor to further challenge the core muscles.

Teaching Tips

Participants may try to place the body in the most challenging or advanced position before they are ready for it. This action will lead to poor technique and positioning because they will not have the strength to perform the exercise properly. Remember that the abdominal muscles must be engaged to maintain a stable core throughout the exercise. Participants should perform the exercise only to the degree to which they can control the movement and maintain the desirable core position.

Props

None.

9. SCISSORS

Goal

Train the pelvis, abdominal muscles, and rib cage to work in unison during a movement, and increase hamstring muscle flexibility.

Initial Positioning

Lie down on your back and lift one leg extended straight out and held just off of and parallel with the floor, and lift the other leg extended straight up toward the ceiling. Lift the upper torso up off the mat by pulling the rib cage in toward the pelvis.

Movement Components and Breathing

Inhale and reach out with both hands to move the leg closer to the chest. Exhale and alternate the position of the legs, lowering one and raising the other, all the while maintaining the arm position and contraction in the torso. Inhale and switch legs again. One cycle of breathing equals one repetition. Repeat the cycle three to five times.

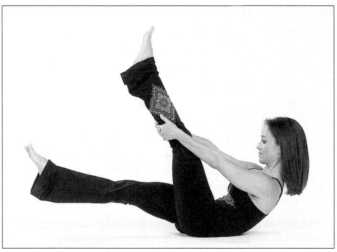

Verbal Cueing Suggestions

- "Keep a neutral spine."
- "Contract the abdominal muscles and rib cage."
- "Keep the neck long, in a neutral position."

Modifications

- Novice: Keep the hands behind the head and the legs slightly bent.
- Advanced: Move the lower leg further down toward the floor with each repetition.

Teaching Tips

Remind participants to focus on each one of the individual components of the movement: the core positioning and stabilization, the leg movement, and the arm position. Remind them to keep all of the muscles engaged throughout the movement.

Props

None.

10. SPINE STRETCH

Goal

Increase thoracic mobility and articulate the spine.

Initial Positioning

Sit upright with the legs extended out straight on the mat, separated hip-width apart. Reach the arms out toward the feet, parallel with the legs, shoulder-width apart.

Movement Components and Breathing

Inhale, keeping the rib cage and the abdominal muscles engaged, the shoulders down and back, and the neck extended long. Exhale and begin to bend forward, as if peeling the spine down one vertebra at a time, with the arms reaching forward. Keep the head in neutral alignment as you bend forward and down, with flexion occurring at the thoracic vertebrae or mid-spine. Inhale and lift back up to the starting position. Repeat the movement three to five times.

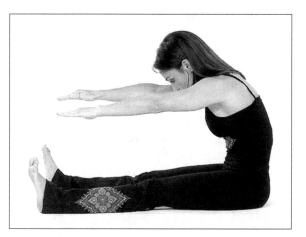

Verbal Cueing Suggestions

- "Pretend you are sitting tall against a wall. Peel the spine off the wall, but don't allow the hips to move. Then roll the spine back up against the wall."
- "Keep a neutral spine. Don't move the hips."
- "As you reach forward, contract the abdominal muscles and lower the spine one vertebra at a time."
- "As you come back up, contract the abdominal muscles and raise the spine one vertebra at a time."
- "Keep the feet flexed and the legs straight."

Modifications

Novice: Sit with the back against a wall. Limit the ROM to the point just before the pelvis begins to move.

Teaching Tips

Beginning participants may not have the flexibility to sit upright with proper posture. If this is the case, have them sit on a pillow or book to help them assume and maintain the proper posture. You can also have participants sit back to back with a partner.

Props

None.

11. LEG LOWERS

Goal

Develop stabilization of the pelvis and rib cage.

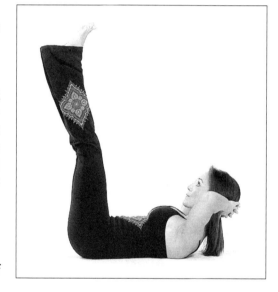

Initial Positioning

Lie down on your back with the neck extended long. Lift the upper torso by contracting the abdominal muscles, bringing the rib cage toward the pelvis. Lift both legs up straight toward the ceiling, keep them together, and place the hands behind the head with the elbows out wide.

Movement Components and Breathing

Maintaining the contraction and position of the torso, inhale and lower both legs straight toward the floor, but not touching the floor. Exhale and raise the legs back up. Repeat the movement three to five times.

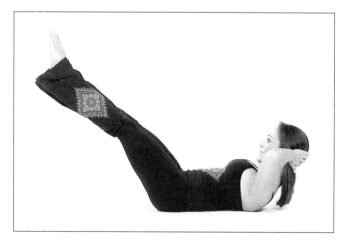

Verbal Cueing Suggestions

- "Contract the abdominal muscles." (This protects the lower back and maintains neutral alignment of the spine and pelvis.)
- "Keep a neutral spine."
- "Lower the legs only as far as you can without lifting your back up off of the mat."

Modifications

- Novice: Keep the head and shoulders resting on the mat and perform the rest of the movement as described earlier. A second modification is to start with the knees bent and the lower legs parallel to the floor. From this position, lower the toes toward the floor, maintaining the bent-knee position throughout the movement. Reduce movement range of motion.
- Advanced: Lower the legs further down toward the floor, maintaining spinal and hip stabilization.

Teaching Tips

Assure participants that there is value in doing this exercise even if they can only slightly lower the legs down toward the floor. You may have to remind beginning participants that this will help them strengthen the core muscles to eventually enable them to maximize this movement. Note that this exercise is sometimes called *Double-Leg Lower Lift*.

Props

- Magic Circle: Place the Magic Circle between the ankles and hold it in place by engaging the muscles of the inner thighs.
- Flat resistance band: Tie the band around the soles of the feet, and hold the ends of the band in the hands.

12. ROCKING

Goal

Utilize the strength of the core muscles along with overall flexibility to perform a movement that is both fun and beneficial.

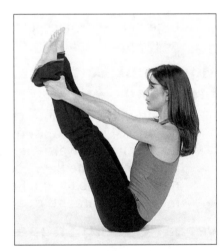

Initial Positioning

Sit at the front edge of the mat with the knees drawn in toward the chest, holding the feet off the floor and with the hands holding on to the legs under the knees.

Movement Components and Breathing

Exhale and begin lifting the body into a more upright position, keeping the shoulders back and down, the neck extended, and the rib cage and abdominal muscles engaged. Straighten out the legs, keeping the knees together and the hands on the legs as you balance the entire body on the sit bone in a V position, all the time maintaining the integrity of the torso. Inhale, curl the chin toward the chest, and let the body rock back onto the shoulder blades, keeping this same body position. Exhale and roll back up to the seated position. Do three repetitions with the feet together and three with the feet apart.

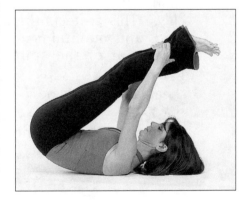

Verbal Cueing Suggestions

- "Contract the abdominal muscles and rib cage, keep the shoulders back and down, and extend the neck." (This position must be maintained throughout the movement.)
- "Stop rolling back when the shoulder blades contact the mat." (This avoids placing undue pressures on the neck and head.)
- "Engage your back and hamstring muscles to control your rocking."

Modifications

- Novice: Place the hands behind the knees and bend the knees. Limit the range of the rocking motion so that you do not jeopardize the stabilization of the torso.
- Advanced: Place the hands on the ankles and fully extend the legs.

Teaching Tips

Because rolling momentum can be a factor in this movement, it is important to keep the focus on trunk stabilization and limit the ROM until the participant develops greater strength. Note that this exercise is sometimes called *Open-Leg Rocker.*

Props

Flat resistance band (advanced only): Place the band on the soles of the feet and hold on to the ends of the band during the movement.

13. CORKSCREW

Goal

Strengthen the oblique muscles of the trunk and enhance core stabilization during movement of the lower body.

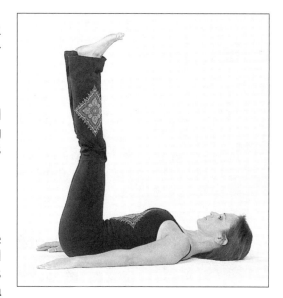

Initial Positioning

Lie down on your back with both legs held together and extended up toward the ceiling at a 90-degree angle to the floor, the arms resting on the mat alongside the body.

Movement Components and Breathing

Start by holding the feet together at the heels, engaging the core muscles, and contracting the muscles of the inner thighs to keep the legs together. Inhale and draw a circle with the legs by moving them together to one side of the body, around, and then exhale and bring the legs back to the starting position. Repeat the movement, circling the legs to the other side. This is one cycle; repeat the cycle three to five times.

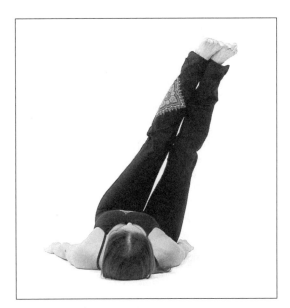 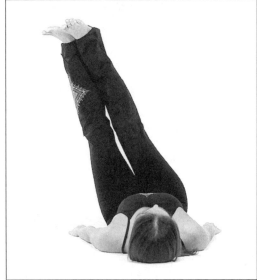

Verbal Cueing Suggestions

- "Contract the abdominal muscles and rib cage, keep the shoulders back and down, and extend the neck." (This position must be maintained throughout the movement.)
- As participants move the legs to the sides, remind them to "Keep a neutral spine and keep the hips on the floor."
- "Pull the shoulders back and down. Press the arms into the mat for support."
- "Keep the feet together at the heels." (They must stay this way throughout the movement.)

Modifications

- Novice: Limit the movement ROM if unable to maintain torso stabilization.
- Advanced: Lift the hips off of the floor so that the body is supported on the shoulders. From here, turn the hips to one side and lower the spine back down to the floor one vertebra at a time. From this new position, draw a circle with the legs in the opposite direction of the hip turn. Then pull the body back up to resting on the shoulders again, and repeat on the opposite side.

Teaching Tips

During the advanced modification of this move, participants will need to exert more force with their core muscles to provide the greater degree of core stabilization needed to maintain the body's stability throughout the movement.

Props

None.

14. SAW

Goal

Train the body to twist at the mid-thoracic spine without moving the hips, a movement that will assist in removing air from the lungs during exhalation.

Initial Positioning

Sit with the legs extended out straight on the mat and spread them more than hip-width apart, feet neutral. Hold the arms out to the sides and parallel to the floor at shoulder height.

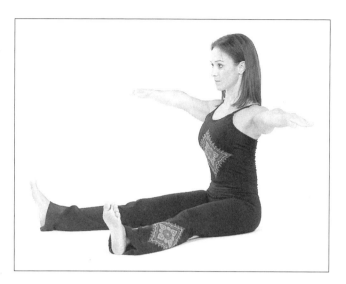

Movement Components and Breathing

Sitting upright with the chest lifted, the shoulders back and down, and the rib cage and abdominal muscles engaged, inhale and begin to turn the torso to one side. Exhale and bend forward, reaching toward the foot on that side with the hand of the opposite arm. Reach with the fingers toward the outside edge of the foot, while the other arm aims behind you, with the palm facing up. Inhale and return to the starting position.

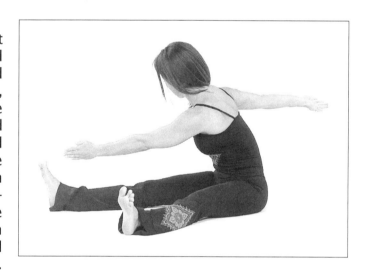

Repeat the movement to the other side. This is one cycle; repeat the cycle four to six times.

Verbal Cueing Suggestions

- "Keep the pelvis and the abdominal muscles contracted throughout the movement."
- As the students twist and reach toward the foot, say, "Exhale fully before you return the torso to center."
- During the twist, say, "Reach from your spine without moving the pelvis." (Avoid bending the spine to reach toward the foot.)

Modifications

Novice: You can sit on a pillow or book to elevate the hips which will help to maintain proper posture in the torso and pelvis. You can also perform the movement with the knees slightly bent. Another option is to keep the arms folded in front of and against your body.

Teaching Tips

Remind participants not to focus their energies on touching the toes. Doing so will cause participants, particularly beginners, to bend at the waist and move the pelvis out of position. The pelvis is not involved in the twist or the reach—the reach comes from the mid-thoracic spine. Maintaining proper postural position is more important than actually reaching the toes.

Props

None.

modified.

15. SWAN

Goal

Engage the erector spinae muscles of the trunk.

Initial Positioning

Lie on your front with the legs extended together straight out on the mat, and the head facing straight down into the mat. This exercise is from a front-lying position, so you need to pay particular attention to body alignment, because you have been accustomed to aligning the body in a back-lying position. Although you feel different when lying facedown, the alignment principles are the same: Make sure that the shoulders are back and down, the spine is neutral, and the abdominal muscles are contracted.

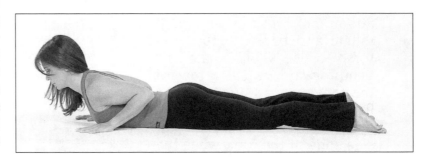

Movement Components and Breathing

Place the palms of the hands on the floor just below the shoulders, with the elbows bent. Inhale and press the shoulder blades down. Exhale and slowly lift the upper body up by first lifting with the spine and then pressing with the arms a bit more without releasing the abdominal and pelvic muscles. Inhale and lower the body back down to the starting position. Repeat the movement three to five times.

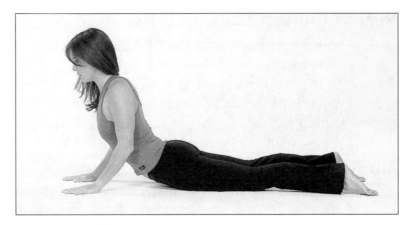

Verbal Cueing Suggestions

- "Contract the abdominal muscles and stabilize the rib cage." (This will help protect the lower back.)
- "Keep your weight on the hips."
- "Press the thighs and heels together, and keep the toes turned out."
- "Keep the neck long, in a neutral position."
- During the lift, say, "Don't throw your head back."

Keep Abs & pelvis on floor.

Modifications

- Novice: Limit the movement range of motion to only what you can do while maintaining torso alignment.

Teaching Tips

Remind participants that the lift comes from a combined effort of the rib cage, and the abdominal and erector muscles. Engaging all involved muscle groups will help to protect the spine throughout the movement.

Props

Stability ball: The Swan movement can be simulated with the use of a stability ball. Lie facedown on the ball with the ball resting under the chest and the hands flat on the floor, shoulder-width apart. Engage the hips and lift the legs off the mat, and then lower them to the starting position, coordinating the breath with the movement as described earlier. Following three to four repetitions of this movement, shift the weight of the body on to the feet, maintaining the ball under the chest and the hands on the floor. Keeping the neck in a neutral position and looking directly into the mat, lift the upper body off the ball in a peeling motion, then lower and return to the starting position.

16. SINGLE-LEG KICK

Goal

Maintain upper body and core muscle contraction while lengthening the muscles of the legs.

Initial Positioning

Lie on the front of the body with the upper body lifted and propped up, resting on the forearms and elbows, the legs extended straight out, and the inner thighs engaged, holding the legs together.

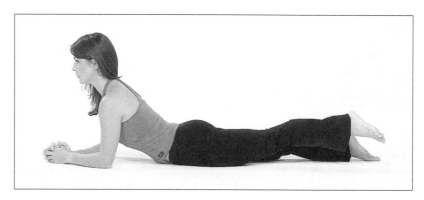

Movement Components and Breathing

Before beginning, make sure that the shoulders are back and down, the spine is in a neutral position, the abdominal muscles are contracted, and the pelvis and hips are in contact with the mat. Inhale and, bending at the knee, kick one leg toward the buttocks two times. Exhale and fully extend the leg, returning it to the starting position on the mat. Alternate legs to complete one cycle of the movement. Repeat the cycle three to five times.

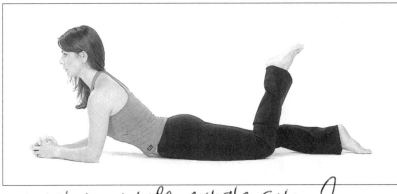

→ Inhale - Inhale - exhale Extend.

Verbal Cueing Suggestions

- As participants are resting on the forearms and elbows to hold the bodies up, remind them, "Keep the shoulders back and down and the chest lifted."
- "Keep the rib cage muscles contracted tightly." (Participants might allow the rib cage to expand as an attempt to make the movement easier to perform.)
- Just before participants begin kicking the legs up, say, "Don't move the hips as you kick."
- When participants exhale after kicking the leg, say, "Extend and lift the leg, then return it to the mat."

Modifications

Novice: Instead of having the upper body lifted and propped up resting on the forearms and elbows, keep the upper body flat on the mat with the forehead resting on the hands.

Teaching Tips

Make sure that participants maintain the integrity of the torso to avoid hyperextension of the spine. Also, remind participants to keep the navel pulled in toward the spine.

Props

Stability ball: Lie facedown on the ball with the ball resting under the chest just above the thighs and place the hands on the mat, shoulder-width apart. Engaging the hips, lift the legs so they are parallel to the floor. Proceed from this position and perform the movement as described earlier.

17. DOUBLE-LEG KICK

Goal

Strengthen the hamstring and gluteal muscles and extend the spine.

Initial Positioning

Lie on your front with the legs extended straight out and together, the hands together behind the back with the elbows bent and the head turned to one side.

Movement Components and Breathing

Before starting the movement, pull the shoulders down and back, contract the rib cage and the abdominal muscles, and maintain a neutral spine. Inhale and exhale, then kick both legs toward the buttocks three times, bending at the knees. After the third kick, from the bent-knee position, inhale and then extend the legs straight back, holding the feet just off the mat and simultaneously lifting the upper body off the floor, lifting from the chest and raising the arms up slightly off the back and straightening them out. Exhale and return to the starting position, turning the head to the other side. Repeat the sequence three to five times.

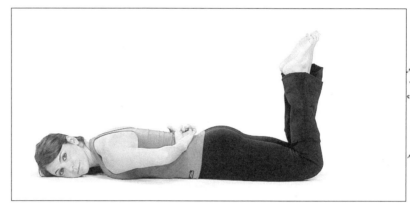

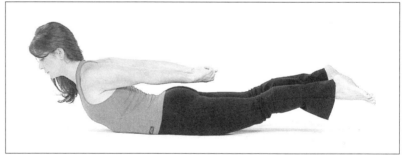

3 kicks then extend.
Turn head R-center then do left.

Verbal Cueing Suggestions

- After each repetition when the participants return to the starting position, say, "Turn your head to the other side."
- When participants lift the upper body off the floor, say, "Extend the arms straight back and lengthen the legs."
- Before starting the movement, remind participants, "Contract the rib cage with the navel toward the spine." (They must stay this way throughout the movement.)
- Just before participants kick the legs up, say, "Don't move the hips as you kick."

Modifications

Novice: Limit the ROM, or eliminate the lifting of the upper body during the second part of the movement.

Teaching Tips

When learning this movement, it is natural for the participants to want to expand the rib cage. Remind them to keep it contracted to control the movement of the spine. Remember that this movement, like many in Pilates, is composed of several small movements—and each of them needs to be emphasized to assure the success of the entire movement.

Props

Stability ball: Lie facedown on the ball with the ball resting under the hips just above the thighs and the hands resting on the mat, shoulder-width apart. Lift the legs up and hold them parallel to the floor by engaging the hips. Proceed from this position to perform the movement as described earlier, but keeping the hands on the mat.

18. BICYCLE TWIST *Cris Cross*

Goal

Strengthen the oblique muscles of the core during trunk rotation while maintaining stability through the hips.

Initial Positioning

Lie down on your back with hands clasped behind your head and lift the head off the mat. Bend the knees in toward the chest and lift both feet off the floor, keeping the lower legs parallel to the floor.

Movement Components and Breathing

Inhale and extend one leg straight out, not letting it touch the floor. At the same time, twist the torso to the opposite side of that leg, aiming the shoulder toward the bent knee. Exhale and switch leg positions, twisting to the other side. One cycle of breathing equals one repetition. Repeat the cycle three to five times.

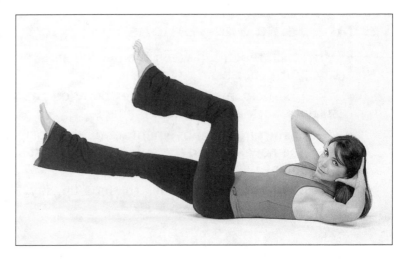

Verbal Cueing Suggestions

- "Keep your leg parallel to the mat as you extend it, and keep the lower portion of the bent leg parallel to the mat."
- "Twist from your spine." (Remind participants to twist the whole torso, not just bend the elbow in toward the knee.)
- "Contract the abdominal muscles and the rib cage." (They must stay this way throughout the movement.)
- "Rest the head in the hands and maintain a neutral spine."

Modifications

Novice: Do not extend the leg straight out; keep the knee somewhat bent.

Teaching Tips

The goal of this exercise is not to have the elbow reach the knee. This is a somewhat complex move, so give continual reminders for each part of the movement. The desire to expand the rib cage will be strong because it will allow for greater rotation. Be sure to correct this when you see it, and remind participants that contracting the ribs and abdominal muscles will help them stay strong and maintain proper positioning. Note that this exercise is sometimes called either *Crisscross* or *Obliques.*

Props

None.

19. THE BRIDGE

Goal

Articulate the spine and strengthen the leg muscles while maintaining hip and pelvic stabilization.

Initial Positioning

Lie down on your back with the knees bent and the feet flat on the mat, hip-width apart, and the arms lying on the mat by the sides.

Movement Components and Breathing

Before beginning, check body positioning and alignment: The neck should be extended long, the shoulders should be back and down, and the rib cage and the abdominal muscles should be engaged. Inhale and begin to lift the hips off the mat so that the shoulder blades bear most of the body weight, articulating through the spine as you lift. Once the hips are elevated, exhale and lift one leg straight up toward the ceiling, then inhale, lower the leg, and bend the knee back to the starting position, returning the foot to the mat. Exhale and perform the same movement with the other leg. Inhale and begin to lower the hips back to the mat, reversing the articulation as you lower down one vertebra at a time. Repeat this cycle three to five times.

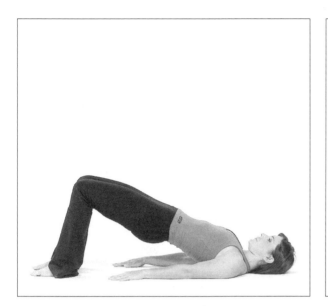
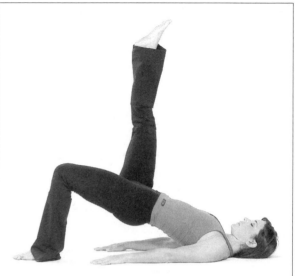
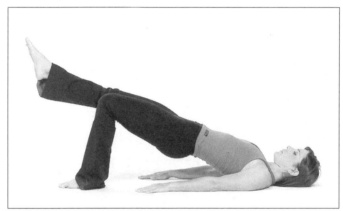

Verbal Cueing Suggestions

- "Lift the back up one vertebra at a time."
- "Lower the back down one vertebra at a time."
- "Keep your weight on the shoulders and shoulder blades."
- "Keep a neutral spine."
- "Engage the rib cage." (They must stay this way throughout the entire movement.)
- "Engage the hip and inner thigh muscles to help stabilize the pelvis."

Modifications

- Novice: On the hip lift component of the movement, reduce the movement ROM only to the point that you can perform the spinal articulation and maintain a neutral spine. For the leg raise component of the movement, rather than try to lift the leg straight up toward the ceiling, pick the foot up only a few inches off the floor. Gradually increase the height of the lift.
- Advanced: When the leg is extended straight up towards the ceiling, instead of bending the knees and returning to the starting position, lower the straight leg toward the floor; then bend it back to the starting position.

Teaching Tips

In performing this movement the first few times, participants will often rush through the process of spinal articulation and lose their focus of moving through each vertebrae. You will need to remind participants to keep the torso and the hips fully engaged and stabilized throughout the movement.

Props

Stability ball: Have the participants lying on their backs on the mat, with both ankles resting on the ball. From this position, have them perform the bridge movement position as described earlier.

20. SIDE-LEG KICK SERIES

Goal

Develop core muscle stabilization and balance during controlled leg movement.

Initial Positioning

Lie down on one side with the head resting on the outstretched lower arm and the upper arm resting in front of the body, with the hand on the floor.

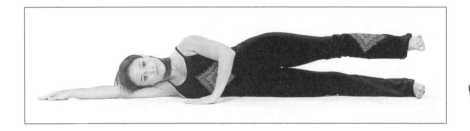

Don't arch Back

Movement Components and Breathing

- Phase One: Before starting the movement, engage the muscles of the torso, make sure that the hips are stacked one on top of the other, and check for a neutral spine. Lift the top leg off the bottom one, then inhale and kick the upper leg forward and out in front of you, keeping the foot flexed and the spine neutral. Exhale and kick the leg back even with the bottom leg but not resting on it, with the toes pointed. Use the upper arm with the hand on the floor to help stabilize the body during the kick. Repeat the movement three to five times; then move to the other side and repeat the movement three to five times again.

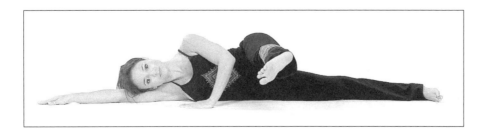

- Phase Two: From the same starting position, perform the kick up and down rather than forward and back, again making sure to maintain the integrity of the torso.

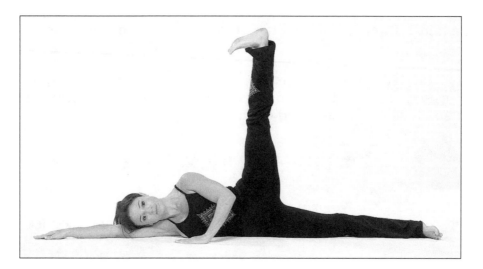

Verbal Cueing Suggestions

- Just before participants kick the leg, say, "Don't move your hips as you kick."
- "Keep a neutral spine."

Modifications

- Novice: Limit the movement ROM so as not to compromise the integrity of the torso.

Teaching Tips

When first learning this movement, participants may try to use some hip movement to make the kick larger. Remind them that the distance of the kick is not as important as maintaining stability of the hips and the torso while the leg is in motion.

Props

None.

21. SEAL

Goal

Strengthen the core, develop balance and coordination, and massage the muscles of the spine.

Initial Positioning

Sit on the front of the mat with the knees bent and the feet off the ground, balancing on the sit bones with the arms reaching between the thighs and then under the lower legs and the hands grasping the outsides of the ankles. Tuck the elbows into the thighs to engage the triceps muscles, helping to maintain stability.

Movement Components and Breathing

Before starting the movement, contract the abdominal muscles and lower the ribs toward the pelvis to allow the spine to become rounded. Inhale, clap the feet together three times, and let the body roll back on the mat, maintaining the same body position and stopping before the shoulders and neck touch the mat. Exhale and roll up to the starting position and again clap the feet together three times. Repeat the cycle three to five times.

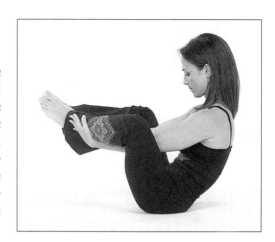

Verbal Cueing Suggestions

- "Contract the rib cage and abdominal muscles." (They must stay this way throughout the movement.)
- As participants are rolling back, say, "Stop" when they reach the lower ridge of the scapula to avoid any undue pressure on the neck and shoulders.
- "Pull the chin in toward the chest." (The participants must maintain this position throughout the movement.)

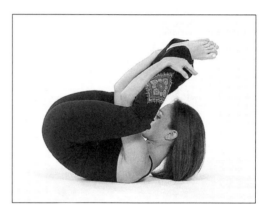

Modifications

- Novice: Limit the movement ROM as you are rolling back.
- Advanced: Deepen the breath and increase the rhythm of the movement slightly.

Teaching Tips

Be aware that momentum may cause participants to exceed the recommended range of the movement. Remind participants to focus on the components of the movement by precisely cueing each phase of the movement. This will help them to better control the rolling motion.

22. NECK PULL

Goal

Articulate the spine, strengthen the core muscles, and stretch the hamstrings.

Initial Positioning

Lie down on your back with the legs extended straight out on the mat, separated hip-width apart. Clasp the hands behind the head.

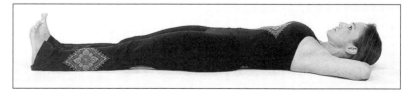

Movement Components and Breathing

Take a breath in and out, contracting the muscles of the lower body to help secure them to the mat. Bring the chin in toward the chest, contract the core muscles to bring the rib cage toward the pelvis, and slowly roll the body up through a sitting position, peeling the spine off the mat during the lifting, continuing forward over the thighs and rounding the back. Inhale and bring the body back to a straight-sitting position of 90 degrees. Exhale and scoop the belly, tuck the pelvis, and roll the body back down to the starting position. Repeat the cycle three to five times.

Verbal Cueing Suggestions

- "Roll up one vertebra at a time."
- "Roll down one vertebra at a time."
- "Engage the rib cage and abdominal muscles and the hamstrings when lowering the spine."

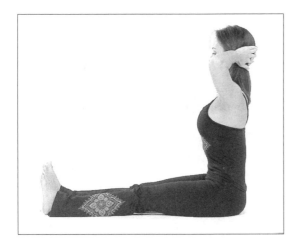 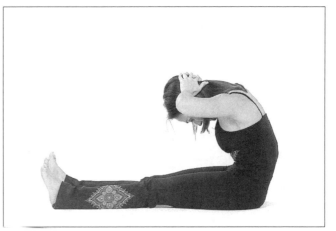

Modifications

Novice: Limit the movement ROM. Also, keep the arms on the mat by the sides of the body with palms facing toward the ceiling, and have the knees bent with the feet flat on the mat.

Teaching Tips

Watch that participants don't pull on the neck with the hands. Instruct participants to utilize the muscles of the core and lower body to perform the movement in a safe and fluid manner. In addition, remind them to keep the shoulders back to avoid excess forces against the neck.

Props

None.

23. SPINE TWIST

Goal

Activate the core muscles and enhance flexibility of the spine with rotation.

Initial Positioning

Sit with the legs extended straight out, the feet together and flexed, and the arms held straight out to the sides from the shoulders.

Movement Components and Breathing

Before beginning the movement, inhale and lift the chest, keeping the shoulders down and back with the abdominal muscles and rib cage contracted. Exhale and rotate the body to one side without bending the upper body, moving primarily from the spine without any movement in the hips or legs. Exhale a second time and rotate a bit further. Inhale, lengthen the spine, and then return to the starting position. Repeat the movement, this time turning to the other side. Perform the cycle three to five times.

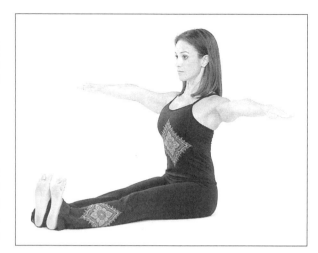

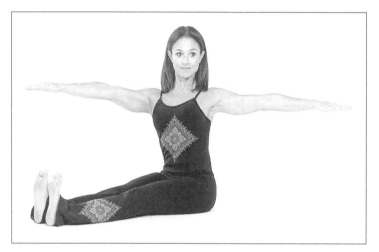

Verbal Cueing Suggestions

- "Pull the shoulders down and back, and contract the abdominal muscles and rib cage."
- "Keep the spine long; imagine there is a string at the top of the head that is gently pulling you up."
- "Twist from the spine." (The hips should not move.)
- "Press the thighs together so that they don't move as you are twisting."

Modifications

Novice: Reduce the movement ROM to match the beginning participants' abilities. One way to help maintain core stability is to have participants sit with the legs bent and crossed at the ankles. In addition, participants can place a book or pillow under the hips if they feel tightness in the lower back or hamstring muscles.

Teaching Tips

You will need to remind the participants to activate the core muscles as they are rotating the spine, and not just to focus on the rotation. You should emphasize the separate components of the twist and not just the whole movement.

Props

None.

24. JACKKNIFE

Goal

Develop strength in the core muscles while stretching the back and shoulders.

Initial Positioning

Lie down on your back with the arms resting on the mat by the sides of the body and the legs extended straight up toward the ceiling perpendicular to the floor.

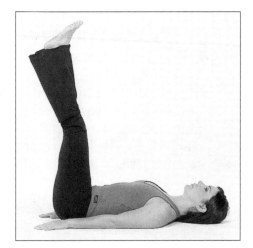

Movement Components and Breathing

Before starting, check for correct positioning: Lengthen the neck, pull the shoulders down and back, and contract the rib cage and abdominal muscles. Inhale and exhale; then begin to elevate the legs higher up to the ceiling, peeling the spine off of the mat one vertebra at a time. When legs are fully extended, you will be balancing on the shoulders. Inhale and begin to lower the hips, peeling the spine down one vertebra at a time, and return the hips to the floor. Repeat the cycle three to five times.

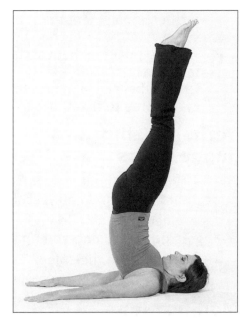

Verbal Cueing Suggestions

- Throughout the lifting and lowering phases of the movement, say, "Contract the abdominal muscles and rib cage."
- As participants lift the legs up, say, "Press the arms down into the mat."
- "Press the thighs together so that they don't move."

Modifications

Novice: Limit the movement ROM based on the abilities of the beginning participants. Rather than have participants try to hold the legs straight up while balancing on the shoulders, have them lower the legs over the head bringing them closer to the floor. From there, they can reverse the movement and lower the hips back to the floor.

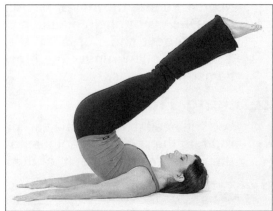

Teaching Tips

Instructors should be aware that the Jackknife is a more advanced move, and participants should master the Roll-Over before attempting it. In order to raise the legs at the start of the movement, participants may be tempted to use the arms much more than the abdominal muscles. Remind them to focus on engaging the abdominal muscles, which will help alleviate stress on the spine as the legs are lifted off the floor. In addition, remind participants to articulate the spine and not just drop the hips as they lower the legs back to the floor.

Props

None.

25. TEASER PREP

Goal

Fully engage and use the strength of the core muscles.

Initial Positioning

Lie down on your back with the arms lying on the mat by your sides, the legs bent at the knees, and the feet flat on the floor.

Movement Components and Breathing

Before starting the movement, check that the neck is extended, the shoulders are back and down, and the rib cage is engaged. Inhale and exhale; then lift the upper body off the floor, contracting the abdominal muscles and articulating the spine with the arms reaching toward the legs. At the same time as the upper body is lifting, raise one foot off the floor and straighten out that leg, holding the knees together tightly. Inhale and exhale, lower the upper body back to the starting position, and lower the straight leg back to the starting position. Repeat the movement, this time lifting and straightening the other leg. Repeat the movement two to three times with each leg.

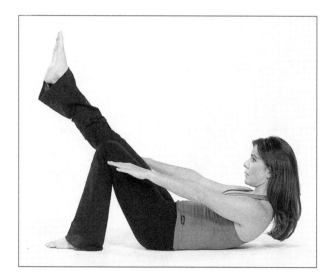 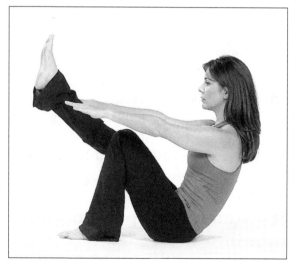

Verbal Cueing Suggestions

- "Pull the shoulders down and back, contract the rib cage and the abdominal muscles, and lengthen the neck." (They must stay this way throughout the movement.)
- As participants raise the upper body, say, "Roll up one vertebra at a time."

Modifications

- Novice: Only lift the upper body off the floor, and have no movement in the lower body; keep the knees bent with both feet flat on the floor throughout the movement. As strength develops, you may progress to lifting one foot off the floor, keeping the other knee bent.

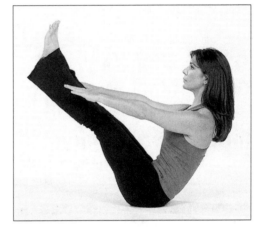

- Advanced: In the initial position, extend the legs straight out on the mat instead of bending them at the knees. Then lift the upper body as described earlier, at the same time lifting both legs up straight so the body is in a V position. Hold, then roll the spine back to the mat, and lower the legs to the starting position. This advanced modification is a slight variation of the classic Teaser exercise.

Teaching Tips

Because this is a somewhat complex movement that uses all the muscles of the core, you will need to precisely cue every phase of the movement, almost as if each were a separate movement.

Props

Magic Circle: Place the Magic Circle between the hands and press inward with the hands to hold it in place to engage the muscles of the upper torso.

26. HIP CIRCLES

Goal

Develop upper body stabilization during lower body movement.

Initial Positioning

Sit on the mat and lean back, resting on the elbows; then hold the legs together and off the mat, straight up in the air at a 90-degree angle from the torso, so the body is in a V position.

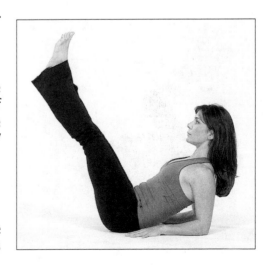

Movement Components and Breathing

Before starting the movement, make sure that the chest is uplifted with the shoulders back and down, and the neck is lengthened. Keeping the rib cage engaged and abdominal muscles contracted, inhale and make a circle with the legs over one side, keeping them together and straight. Exhale and circle the legs to the other side. Repeat the movement three to five times on each side.

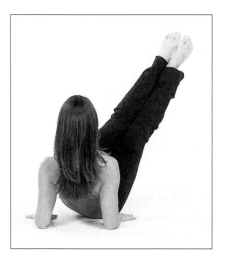

Verbal Cueing Suggestions

- "Pull the shoulders down and back, contract the abdominal muscles and rib cage, and lengthen the neck." (They must stay this way throughout the movement.)
- "Keep the chest lifted." (This maintains the length in the spine.)
- "Keep the upper body still."
- "Keep the neck long and in a neutral position."

Modifications

- Novice: Limit the movement ROM, and bend the knees slightly as the legs circle.
- Advanced: In the initial position, instead of leaning back on the elbows, extend the arms fully to support the upper body, placing the hands flat on the floor. From this position, be sure to maintain the arm muscle engagement so they can assist in controlling unwanted movement of the torso.

Teaching Tips

Be aware that when first learning this movement, participants may let the chest sink down, making it a bit easier to circle the legs. Remind participants that the objective is to engage all the core muscles, and they may need to reduce the movement range of motion to maintain core stability.

Props

None.

27. SWIMMING

Goal

Strengthen the muscles along the spinal column.

Initial Positioning

Lie on your front with the head facing straight down and in alignment, arms stretched out overhead with the hands on the floor, and the legs extended straight back, also resting on the floor. Spread both the arms and the legs approximately shoulder-width apart.

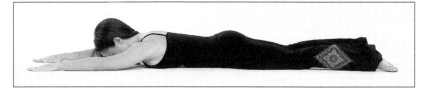

Movement Components and Breathing

Before starting the movement, make sure that the neck is lengthened, and the rib cage and abdominal muscles are contracted and engaged. Inhale and lift the head, looking straight down into the floor, and raise one arm and the opposite leg, extending them out straight and off the floor. Exhale, lowering the arm and the leg, still holding them off the floor. Inhale and raise the other arm and leg. Repeat the lowering and lifting of the opposite sides three to five times so the movement resembles a controlled swimming motion.

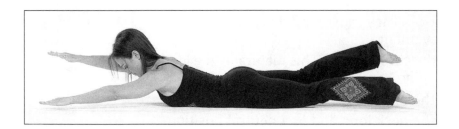

Verbal Cueing Suggestions

- "Contract the abdominal muscles." (This will help prevent hyperextension during the movement.)
- As participants lift the head, remind them, "Keep the neck long."

Modifications

- Novice: Limit the movement ROM, not lifting the arms and legs too high.
- Advanced: Start by lifting the upper torso, arms, and both legs off the floor. Keep the head facing down, and maintain that position. From there, proceed to lift one arm and the opposite leg a bit higher as you inhale, and then lift the other arm and leg as you exhale. Participants can create a rhythm of movement with the breath by inhaling for 5 counts of movement, and then exhaling for 5 counts of movement.

Teaching Tips

Because of all the movement in this exercise, participants may lose focus on contracting and engaging the rib cage and abdominal muscles, which will allow the rib cage to open up during the movement. Remind them to check these muscles and maintain stability to protect the spine and allow the erector muscles to contract without undue pressure on the vertebrae.

Props

None.

28. LEG PULL FRONT

Goal

Develop upper body strength and core stability.

Initial Positioning

Get into a full push-up position with the body facing the mat, legs extended, up on the toes, the arms straight, and the hands on the floor directly under the shoulders.

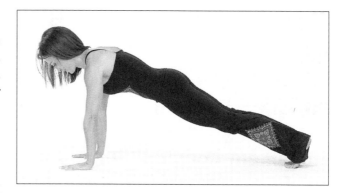

Movement Components and Breathing

Before starting the movement, make sure that the rib cage and abdominal muscles are contracted and engaged and the spine is neutral. Inhale and lift one leg up off the floor, extending it out from the hip. Only lift the foot as high as the head. From a side view, there should be a straight line from the crown of the head to the heel of the foot. Exhale and lower the leg. Repeat the movement with the other leg. Repeat the movement three to five times on each leg.

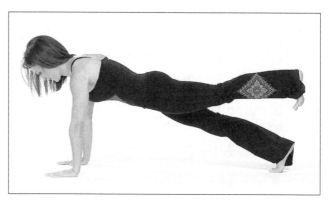

Verbal Cueing Suggestions

- "Contract the rib cage and abdominal muscles." (They must stay this way throughout the movement.)
- "Keep the head facing down and the neck long." (They must stay this way throughout the movement.)
- As participants lift their leg, say, "Extend your leg back and away from the hip. Keep your other leg and hip still."

Modifications

- Novice: Perform the movement with the arms bent, so that the body is propped up on the elbows instead of the hands.
- Advanced: Work on increasing movement ROM without compromising form, stability, and technique.

Teaching Tips

As with all of the Pilates movements, it is important to remind participants to focus on each of the integral parts of the movement, and not just on the movement as a whole. Also, be aware that the spine will sag and the hips will move excessively if the core muscles are not properly engaged.

Props

Stability ball: Have participants lie facedown on the ball with both hands on the floor shoulder-width apart and both feet on the floor. The ball should rest between the abdomen and the thighs. From this position, perform the movement as stated earlier.

29. THE PUSH-UP

Goal

Develop upper body strength and core muscle stability.

Initial Positioning

Stand with torso straight and the arms extended overhead.

Movement Components and Breathing

Before starting the movement, make sure that the rib cage and abdominal muscles are engaged. Inhale, exhale, and slowly bend forward, peeling the spine down with the arms reaching toward the floor. Inhale and begin to walk the hands out away from the feet. Exhale and continue walking the hands out until they are directly under the shoulders and the body is in a push-up position. In this position, the body should be in a straight line from the crown of the head to the heel of the foot. Inhale and lower the body toward the floor, bending the arms; then exhale and return back up. Repeat the push-up two to three times, then walk the hands back toward the feet, and lift the body back up to standing, again peeling the spine.

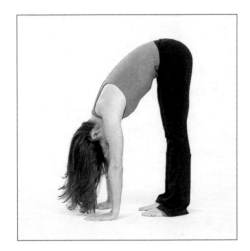
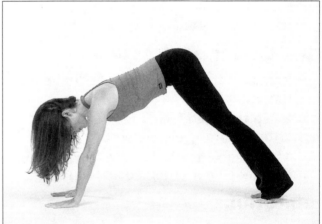
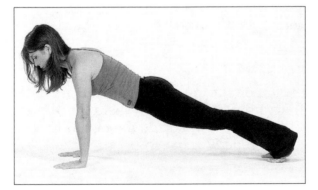
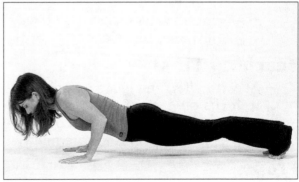

Verbal Cueing Suggestions

- "Contract the rib cage and abdominal muscles." (They must stay this way throughout the movement.)
- "Keep the head facing down and the neck long." (They must stay this way throughout the movement.)
- As participants perform the push-up, remind them, "Keep the elbows tight to the sides."
- "Keep the leg muscles contracted and engaged throughout the movement."

Modifications

- Novice: Start from a kneeling position; this should help you maintain the correct technique and torso stability.
- Advanced: Increase the number of push-up repetitions.

Teaching Tips

Be aware that during the push-up phase, participants may forget to properly engage the core muscles, causing the spine to sag and compromising the stability of the torso.

Props

Stability ball: Lie facedown on the ball with the leg straight and off the floor and the ball resting under the legs anywhere from the thighs (easiest) to the ankles (most challenging). Proceed with the push-up movement as stated earlier.

YMCA Pilates Program Design

Now that all of the exercises have been described to you in detail, you can begin to put them together in a class structure. The YMCA Pilates mat exercise program presents the exercises in three suggested series for instructors to follow in developing different level classes. The 29 exercises, their various modifications, and the occasional use of props can now be combined into a variety of Pilates mat exercise classes. The Pilates mat exercises will never significantly change from the original series of movements, but the sequences, the number of repetitions, and the choices of which modifications and props may be used, may vary from class to class. You may add a move or vary the modification, but the initial movement will always remain the same.

Before teaching a class, you must spend a significant amount of time practicing the exercises to master them with your own body. This practice will enable you not only to better describe and explain the movement to participants, but also to better be able to spot technique mistakes and offer corrective suggestions. In addition, you should continue to be a Pilates student, attending additional classes, workshops, and training events to better understand the exercises and develop your own skills, as well as to learn modifications, specialized techniques, and the use of different exercise props.

As you become more familiar with the movements, you will begin to recognize how they flow from one to the next, and how the entire muscular system is used during each series. When first learning Pilates exercise, the natural tendency is to focus strictly on technique and form, not being too concerned with movement-to-movement flow. With practice, you will become accomplished at maintaining this flow of movements so that it will become easier to teach participants how to move seamlessly through the workout session and have a fulfilling exercise experience. As you and your participants all gain exercise mastery, the most noticeable change in the class will not be in the series of exercises per se, but in the smoothness and continuity of movement. At this point, the class will have evolved from performing a somewhat disconnected series of individual exercises to performing a continual, connected flow of movement for the entire class time.

As you practice and become more familiar with all the Pilates mat exercises presented here, it will become easier to recognize when to incorporate some of the modifications or props to assist the participants' learning of a movement. In doing so, you may find it necessary to vary the sequence of movements a bit. Your goal should be to help participants develop the skills and master each movement. Your own understanding of the movements will make it easier to customize movements to assist each of your participants in reaching their goals.

The following section provides a listing of the exercises in each of the three Pilates mat work sequences: Mat Work 1, 2, and 3. The instructor can use these three sequences as class structure. In addition, the section has suggested formats for an intermediate-level and an advanced-level class.

Pilates Mat Work 1

The 11 Pilates mat exercises in the following list comprise a novice-level Pilates class. Beginning participants will gain a better understanding of the Pilates philosophy, as well as posture and alignment, with these initial movements. Only after all of these movements have been fully mastered should participants move on to Pilates Mat Work 2. Keep in mind that progression rates will vary among participants, and this may take anywhere from a few weeks to a few months.

The warm-up exercises for Pilates Mat Work 1 include

- deep abdominal breathing,
- neutral spine and spinal imprinting,
- retraction, and
- abdominal crunch.

The exercises for Pilates Mat Work 1 include

- the Hundred,
- Assisted Roll-Up,
- Single-Leg Circle,
- Rolling,
- Single-Leg Stretch,
- Double-Leg Stretch,
- Spine Stretch,
- Swan,

- the Bridge,
- Side Kick—Up and Down, and
- Seal.

Pilates Mat Work 2

The 13 Pilates mat exercises in the following list comprise Pilates Mat Work 2, which can be considered a second-stage, novice-level class. This sequence will be the final phase of learning before moving on to an intermediate-level class, which will be a combination of Pilates Mat Work 1 and Pilates Mat Work 2. You should teach this intermediate-level class only after participants have fully mastered the movements presented in Pilates Mat Work 2.

The warm-up exercises for Pilates Mat Work 2 include

- deep abdominal breathing,
- neutral spine and spinal imprinting,
- retraction, and
- abdominal crunch.

The exercises for Pilates Mat Work 2 include

- the Hundred,
- Roll-Up,
- Roll-Over,
- Rolling,
- Scissors,
- Leg Lowers,
- Bicycle Twist,
- Rocking,
- Corkscrew,
- Saw,
- Single-Leg Kick,
- Double-Leg Kick, and
- Side Kick–Front and Back.

Pilates Mat Work: Intermediate-Level Class

The warm-up exercises include

- deep abdominal breathing,
- neutral spine and spinal imprinting,
- retraction, and
- abdominal crunch.

The exercises for the Intermediate-Level class include

- the Hundred,
- Roll-Up,

- Roll-Over,
- Single-Leg Circle,
- Rolling,
- Single-Leg Stretch,
- Double-Leg Stretch,
- Scissors,
- Leg Lowers,
- Bicycle Twist,
- Spine Stretch,
- Rocking,
- Corkscrew,
- Saw,
- Swan,
- Single-Leg Kick,
- Double-Leg Kick,
- the Bridge,
- Side Kick series, and
- Seal.

Pilates Mat Work 3

The 18 Pilates mat exercises in the following list comprise Pilates Mat Work 3, the start of advanced-level Pilates programming. Once all of these movements are mastered, participants may move on to the advanced-level class also listed. As with all Pilates exercises, you will need to do a few more repetitions of the newer advanced movements as participants learn techniques. After that is accomplished, the number of repetitions will decrease. You should encourage participants to focus on perfecting their technique and the precision of each movement. After the advanced techniques have been mastered, the class flow should improve significantly, because participants will not need additional repetitions to learn the beginner and intermediate movements that are incorporated into an advanced-level class.

The warm-up exercises for Pilates Mat Work 3 include

- deep abdominal breathing,
- neutral spine and spinal imprinting,
- retraction, and
- abdominal crunch.

The exercises include

- the Hundred,
- Roll-Up,
- Single-Leg Circle,
- Rolling,
- Spine Stretch,

- Rocking,
- Corkscrew (hips off the ground),
- Swan,
- Neck Pull,
- the Bridge,
- Spine Twist,
- Jackknife,
- Teaser Prep,
- Hip Circles,
- Swimming,
- Leg Pull Front,
- the Push-Up, and
- Seal.

Pilates Mat Work: Advanced-Level Class

The warm-up exercises include

- deep abdominal breathing,
- neutral spine and spinal imprinting,
- retraction, and
- abdominal crunch.

The exercises include

- the Hundred,
- Roll-Up,
- Roll-Over,
- Single-Leg Circle,
- Rolling,
- Single-Leg Stretch,
- Double-Leg Stretch,
- Scissors,
- Leg Lowers,
- Bicycle Twist,
- Spine Stretch,
- Rocking,
- Corkscrew (hips off the ground),
- Saw,
- Swan,
- Single-Leg Kick,
- Double-Leg Kick,
- Neck Pull,

- the Bridge,
- Spine Twist,
- Jack Knife,
- Side Kick series,
- Teaser Prep,
- Hip Circles,
- Swimming,
- Leg Pull Front,
- Seal, and
- the Push-Up.

7

Teaching Pilates Mat Exercise Programs

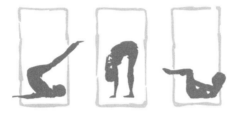

Unlike many traditional group exercise programs, Pilates exercise involves a very detailed type of training that will be new to most participants. Because of the initial learning phase that all beginning Pilates participants go through, it is important for you to create an atmosphere in which participants are comfortable with trying new and perhaps difficult movements. Participants will need to develop trust in your skills to help them learn and grow and to feel successful even in the early stages of the program. If you notice that beginning participants are experiencing difficulty with the exercises and becoming discouraged, you will need to reassure them of the progress they are making. This encouragement will go a long way in motivating them to continue with the program. In your classes, you should create an environment conducive to learning, one that is calmer and perhaps more patient than a traditional group exercise program. Because this type of purposeful exercise requires participants to focus on their own body and its movements, it is truly an individual workout within a group setting. This format provides the opportunity for you to teach each participant how to identify their own personal strengths and weaknesses and how to exercise to best meet their individual needs.

Because of the newness of many Pilates exercises for beginning participants, your ability to communicate directions clearly is one of the most important aspects of a class. Some of the movements in the Pilates mat work series could be considered high risk for some participants if performed incorrectly or mindlessly, so they need a disciplined approach to training. Slow progression and thorough instruction are the key components to teaching a safe and successful Pilates program.

In traditional exercise classes, both participants and instructors often measure success by results such as losing weight, gaining muscle definition, or improving one's strength or endurance. Instructors use external motivational tools such as new, complex movement choreography and exciting, uplifting music to maintain participant interest. A mind–body exercise program such as Pilates is different in this regard, because you measure success by factors such as achieving better awareness of movement and repeating the same movements a number of times to gain mastery. Indeed, regular practice of Pilates exercise will develop greater core muscle strength, produce visible changes in posture, and develop muscular definition. But the philosophical difference is that, with Pilates, those gains are by-products of participants' focusing on movement mastery, rather than focusing on the gains themselves.

Communicating Effectively

Communication is the art of clearly transmitting information to others so that they can receive, review, evaluate, and understand the intended message. People all learn and gain understanding uniquely in that some learn better by seeing, the visual sense; some through listening, the auditory sense; and others still through doing and touching, the tactile sense. These differences can make teaching skills such as Pilates movement more challenging, because you may need to communicate in several ways to get the same point across to a group of people. To become successful at communicating these somewhat complex and different movements to those just starting out, Pilates instructors will need to spend a considerable amount of time practicing not only the movements, but also their ability to give clear directions and verbally describe correct positioning. As your knowledge and understanding of the anatomy, biomechanics, and principles of Pilates movement increases, so will your ability to effectively communicate with participants.

Review Your Communication Skills

Pilates instructors, even experienced ones, should continually review their communication skills to make sure they are fresh and effective. Too many times exercise instructors get comfortable in a particular style, word phrasing, or class routine, and lose focus of the participants' needs. You should periodically review how you are communicating and how your participants perceive you. Following are two techniques to use for this purpose:

1. **Record yourself teaching:** In two different classes, record yourself, first with an audiotape, and then with a videotape. For the first one, set up a tape recorder at the back of the classroom and let it record the entire class. The next day, listen to the entire tape and critique yourself: Did you clearly understand your own instructions? Without seeing the exercises, could you understand precisely how to perform the exercises you described? Then, choose a different class and videotape it from the front of the room, recording the participants as they perform the exercises. You should tell the class why you are recording and ask whether they are comfortable with it. The next day, review the tape: Was everybody performing the exercises correctly? Did it seem that they clearly understood your instructions?

2. **Become a student again.** Attend a few Pilates classes taught by someone else. Participate in the entire class, placing yourself in the back of the room (this is where beginners typically will go). Here is what you should look for:

   - Can you clearly see the movements the instructor is performing?
   - Can you understand the instructions in such a manner that you don't even have to look at the instructor?
   - Do the participants clearly understand all the components of the movement?
   - Did you think that the participants in the class felt successful?
   - Did you feel successful?

Use this information as a learning tool to help you improve your own communication so that your skills as an instructor will grow.

Teaching Tips

Pilates exercise becomes a very personal experience for each participant, so you should approach teaching from a personal perspective with each class member. The following is a list of suggestions to help you in developing individual relationships and effective communications with each participant:

- Learn the names of all your participants.

- Discuss any possible movement limitations or structural deviations with each participant.

- Repeat the instructions for each component of the exercises over and over. Keep in mind that while you may get bored with hearing your own voice repeating the same instructions, participants, particularly beginners trying to master a movement, will welcome this repetition.

- Approach teaching each class with the attitude that you are creating a customized program based on the needs of each particular participant.

- Smile, give ample praise, and make participants feel welcome and successful. This type of positive reinforcement and support will help keep participants motivated and help ensure their continued participation in your program.

- Avoid positioning yourself in one spot in the exercise room. Demonstrate movements in the front of the room to begin a class, but also move around the entire classroom; it is, after all, your teaching space. Moving around the room will allow you not only to view and assist all participants, but also it will give you the opportunity to improve your teaching skills as well, because you will more closely and clearly see whether participants are responding to your verbal instructions.

- Distribute handout information and copies of Pilates-related articles to help participants learn and develop a better understanding of the program. Refer to the many resources listed in the appendix for this type of information

- Teach each component of the movement in detail.

- Maintain the same routine of movements until the participants have fully mastered them.

- Continually emphasize proper alignment and technique.

- Encourage participants to move within their own individual range of motion and work within their own abilities.

- Encourage your class not to concern themselves with how the others are doing, but to focus on their own technique.

- Communicate with a variety of styles, including verbal, visual, and tactile.

- Practice and master the exercises yourself, recognize your imbalances, work on correcting them, and the exercises will become much easier to teach.

Using Music in Pilates Classes

In teaching Pilates exercise, participants should be focusing on the instructor's voice, which should be clear, soothing, and motivating. The use of music in Pilates is strictly for background ambience, not for choreographic purposes as in most traditional group exercise. You should use soft, calming background music that doesn't overstimulate the senses. In this manner, music will work more to assist in soothing the mind and help participants focus on the movements of the body rather than serve to distract them from the movements. The combination of your soothing voice and your appropriately chosen background music will help participants focus on the present moment without undue mental distractions.

Giving Feedback

In Pilates class, your job is not to create variety and style; it is to teach a specific type of movement. As you become more experienced at teaching Pilates classes and working with a wide range of participants, you will become more adept at noticing areas of weakness and postural deviation that need to be corrected. This knowledge will serve you well in correcting participants in a manner that both helps them better understand the movement and makes them feel successful.

After you have described and demonstrated a movement, have participants perform it while you observe them, and give them feedback on their technique. Feedback can be a powerful contributor to effective learning and participant performance. Offer it after participants have asked a question or performed a movement. You can use three types of feedback:

1. **Verbal feedback,** which includes your statements about the participant's performance and your vocal inflections

2. **Nonverbal feedback,** which includes gestures and facial expressions

3. **Guided manipulation,** which is your physical guidance of the participant's body

Giving feedback informs your participants of the correctness of their performance and it recognizes their effort. Your feedback can have a great impact on them.

To give effective feedback, you first must present a clearly defined standard of performance. For example, you define the standard of performance for spinal alignment during a particular movement by explaining and demonstrating it. You and the participants then measure and correct the movement according to the demonstrated criteria. If, after explaining and demonstrating how the spine should be aligned, you notice any deviation, explain the deviation to the participant and then describe how to correct it. Be sure to give the participants time to practice so they can try to correct their performance and reach the preset standard.

Good feedback is specific, is contingent on performance, and provides corrective information for the learner. Specific feedback is clear about what was right or wrong and gives enough information to make necessary adjustments. You may watch a participant incorrectly perform an abdominal crunch and then exclaim, "That's not right!" Such a response does not aid the participant's understanding of the performance; it only lets them know that it was wrong. By contrast, you might respond by explaining, "You need to contract your rib cage toward your pelvis." Such verbal corrective feedback helps the participant know what was wrong with the performance and what to do to get back on track.

Nonverbal feedback can be just as effective as verbal feedback, sometimes even more so. Participants tune in to facial expressions and gestures. When used properly, nonverbal cues are the epitome of personalization. How else can a thumbs-up signal and a generous smile be interpreted? Other nonverbal positive feedback interactions include making an OK sign, nodding, and applauding.

Positive verbal or nonverbal feedback is not needed for every single move, because too much of a good thing can have a negative effect; people tend to disregard excessive compliments. Match your feedback to the achievement and specifically relate your response to the performance.

Use care when you give feedback using guided manipulation—that is, physically touching participants to guide them through a movement. First, describe how you plan to assist them, and ask whether it's OK to touch them. If they agree, tell them where you plan to touch them ("I'm going to place my fingers on your shoulders") and then physically guide them through the desired movement while verbally giving the instructions at the same time. This combination of both guided manipulation and verbal feedback helps participants develop a clear sense of how to perform the correct movement, and it may more easily identify what he or she was doing wrong.

Always use good judgment when providing guided manipulation. Touch participants with a finger or two rather than with your whole hand, and avoid touching any areas of the body that would make you or your participants uncomfortable. If touching isn't possible, because it would make the participant uncomfortable, you can verbally guide participants in using their own hands to assist in performing the movement.

An important point for you to remember regarding feedback is that, as in all interpersonal communication, when you give both verbal and nonverbal feedback, you should try to keep them congruent. For example, if you frown while telling participants that they are doing a great job, the two behaviors are incongruent and the conflicting messages are confusing. Participants may be more likely to believe the frown rather than the words because the visual can be quite powerful. On the other hand, when your feedback is congruent, you can have a powerful positive influence on your participants' reactions.

Addressing Participant Discomfort During Exercise

As the instructor, it is your responsibility to make sure that all participants clearly understand every movement taught in the class so that they can perform it safely and effectively. Having proper control of movement and being aware of posture, alignment, and technique can help participants to avoid most potential discomfort. However, as in any exercise program, some participant discomfort is bound to occur, particularly among beginners. Teaching experience will help you to recognize incorrect movements, misalignments, and poor body placement by participants that, unchecked, could lead to discomfort. There are a number of reasons why Pilates participants may experience discomfort during or after activity. Perhaps they performed a movement incorrectly, or the participants tried something that was beyond what they were ready and capable of doing. Whatever the case, following are two areas of discomfort that are commonly reported by Pilates participants, particularly beginners:

1. **Back pain:** Feeling pain in the back during Pilates exercise most often occurs because participants are not properly and fully contracting the abdominal muscles. In this case, the spine will not have full support during movement, leaving it vulnerable to misalignment. Back pain can also occur if the pelvis is not aligned correctly, which again will result in added forces to the spine. Finally, if the head is not held in the proper position over the cervical vertebrae, the alignment of the spine will be compromised, possibly contributing to discomfort in the back.

2. **Neck pain:** Many of the positions used in Pilates exercise require the neck to sustain a position for an extended period of time. In these positions, the muscles that surround the neck are called on to keep the cervical vertebrae in alignment and hold the neck in place. While proper alignment is important, participants may not have adequate strength in the supporting muscles to avoid neck pain. The particular movement may need to be modified in order for the participant to perform the exercise without discomfort until they have repeated it enough to strengthen the neck muscles.

Common Participant Questions

Following are some questions that new or prospective participants commonly ask about Pilates:

• *What is Pilates?* Pilates is a form of exercise that utilizes the muscles of the body as a whole, instead of working the muscles in isolation as do many traditional exercise programs. It is an exercise system focused on improving flexibility and strength for the total body without building bulk. Pilates is not just exercise, however. It is a series of controlled movements engaging your body and mind, taught by trained instructors.

• *What's the difference between Pilates and Yoga?* In some respects Pilates exercise is like yoga. Both are considered mind–body methods of movement; both emphasize deep breathing and smooth, long movements that encourage your muscles to relax and lengthen. The difference is that, while yoga requires moving from one static posture to the next without repetitions, Pilates flows through a series of movements that are more dynamic, systematic, and anatomically based. The goal with Pilates exercise is to achieve optimal functional fitness.

• *Can you lose weight with Pilates mat classes?* As with any exercise program, you will burn calories, which is one factor in weight loss. But most people who are seeking significant change in body weight will need to supplement additional cardiovascular training or reduce caloric consumption.

• *Do I need to use a machine in order to receive the full benefits of the program?* In Pilates, the mat work program is just as beneficial as exercise on Pilates equipment. The machines may work better for a few specific needs, but the mat program will give most participants everything they need to achieve their goals.

• *Will I be able to perform the mat exercises if I am not flexible?* The beauty of the Pilates program is that it teaches individuals how to work within their abilities. Keep in mind that, while having good flexibility is a plus, it is not a prerequisite. And, through regular practice of Pilates, flexibility will improve as the participant progresses.

• *How many classes a week should I attend?* Unlike activities such as strength training, Pilates exercise does not isolate a particular muscle. Therefore, the muscles do not need the same recovery time as they would with isolation exercise. For this reason, some experienced participants practice Pilates every day, but two to three times a week is recommended for beginners.

• *If I have never exercised before, is Pilates a good way to get started?* Pilates is a great way to get started in a fitness program. Pilates progresses at a slow and individually dictated pace, it gives participants a clear awareness of their individual strengths and weaknesses, and it creates a mindful approach to training.

• *I am presently participating in a strength-training program. Can I also participate in Pilates?* Because Pilates realigns your body for correct posture and movement, you can use Pilates prior to strength training to help focus your attention into your body. On the same note, you can train with weights before a Pilates session, then realign the body with Pilates movements, which may also assist in the recovery of the muscles.

Appendix

Related Resources

There are many sources for Pilates equipment and instructor training programs. The following list includes most of the well-known organizations.

Recommended Pilates Product and Training Resources

YMCA of the USA
101 North Wacker Drive
Chicago, IL 60606
Phone: 800-872-9622
Web site: www.ymca.net

The YMCA of the USA offers certification through YMCA Pilates Instructor, an introductory 8-hour training course in Pilates mat exercise for YMCA instructors. Contact the YMCA of the USA Training Services Department for course availability.

Pilates Method Alliance™
P.O. Box 370906
Miami, FL 33137
Phone: 866-573-4945
Web site: www.pilatesmethodalliance.org
E-mail: info@pilatesmethodalliance.org

The Pilates Method Alliance is an international organization dedicated to preserving the legacy of Joseph H. and Clara Pilates. The PMA maintains and advocates nation standards for Pilates education and information. Check the Web site or call for more information.

Physicalmind Institute®
84 Wooster Street, Suite 405
New York, NY 10012
Phone: 800-505-1990 or 212-343-2150
Web site: www.themethodpilates.com
E-mail: info@themethodpilates.com

The Physicalmind Institute offers open instructor training regularly at certifying studios throughout the country. Check the Web site or call for more information.

PowerHouse Pilates™
85 Sichi Hill Road
Eighty Four, PA 15330
Phone: 877-716-4879
Web site: www.phpilates.com

Offers open instructor trainings regularly at training sites in Kona, Hawaii; Pittsburgh, Pennsylvania; Fort Worth, Texas; Chester, New Jersey; and Sacramento, California. Check the Web site or call for more information.

STOTT PILATES™
2200 Yonge Street, Suite 1402
Toronto, Ontario M4S 2C6
CANADA
Phone: 800-910-0001 (toll free from the U.S. and Canada)
Web site: www.stottpilates.com
E-mail: info@stottpilates.com

STOTT PILATES manufactures and sells Pilates equipment and offers a variety of instructor training programs.

Balanced Body® Inc.
8220 Ferguson Avenue
Sacramento, CA 95828
Phone: 800-PILATES (745-2837) (toll free in the U.S. and Canada)
Web site: www.pilates.com
E-mail: info@pilates.com

Balanced Body Inc. manufactures and sells Pilates equipment and offers a variety of instructor training programs.

Peak Pilates
4865 Riverbend Road, Suite 200
Boulder, CO 80301
Phone: 800-925-3674 or 303-998-1531
Web site: www.peakpilates.com

Peak Body Systems manufactures and sells Pilates equipment and offers a variety of instructor training programs.

SPRI Products, Inc.
1600 Northwind Boulevard
Libertyville, IL 60048
Phone: 800-222-7774
Web site: www.spriproducts.com
E-mail: teamspri@spriproducts.com

SPRI Products, Inc. manufactures and distributes exercise mats, rubberized resistance exercise products, educational materials, instructional manuals and videos, and other fitness equipment and accessories.

Recommended Reading

Calais-Germain, Blandine. 1993. *Anatomy of Movement.* Seattle: Eastland Press.

Clark, Marci, and Christine Romani-Ruby. 2001. *The Pilates Reformer: A Manual for Instructors.* Tarentum, Pa.: Word Association Publishers.

DeBono, Edward. 1994. *DeBono's Thinking Course.* New York: Facts on File, Inc.

Gazda, George and Frank Asbury. 1995. *Human Relations Development.* Boston: Allyn & Bacon.

Hebert, Michele. 1993. The Breath of Life. *IDEA Today,* 31-33.

Norkin, Cynthia, and Pamela Levangie. 1992. *Joint Structure and Function.* Philadelphia: F.A. Davis Company.

Pervis, Tom. 1998. *Biomechanics. Resistance Training Specialist Manual.* Oklahoma: Focus on Fitness.

Pilates, Joseph H. [1934] 1998. *Your Health: A Corrective System of Exercising that Revolutionizes the Entire Field of Physical Education.* Edited by Judd Robbins. Incline Village, Nev.: Presentation Dynamics Inc.

Pilates, Joseph H., and William J. Miller. 2000. *A Pilates' Primer: The Millennium Edition.* Incline Village, Nev.: Presentation Dynamics Inc.

Pilates, Joseph H., and William J. Miller. [1945] 1998. *Pilates' Return to Life Through Contrology.* Edited by Judd Robbins. Incline Village, Nev.: Presentation Dynamics Inc.

Polestar Education. 2000. *Polestar Rehabilitation Instructor Training Manual.* Coral Gables, Fla.: Polestar Education.

Roane, Susan. 1997. *The Verbal Edge.* New York: Warner Books.

Siler, Brooke. 2000. *The Pilates Body.* New York: Random House, Inc.

Slavin, Mark. 2000. *The Biomechanics of Movement.* Key Biscayne, FL: Professional Fitness, Inc.

Spence, Alexander P., and Elliot B. Mason. 1983. *Human Anatomy and Physiology.* San Francisco: The Benjamin/Cummings Publishing Company.

STOTT PILATES™. 2001. *Comprehensive Matwork Manual.* Toronto, Canada: Merrithew Corp.

Recommended Videotapes for Pilates Instructor Training

Many videotapes are geared for the consumer market and are not created for instructor training purposes. The following videotapes either include a section for teaching techniques or are dedicated entirely to instructor training, and they are listed by vendor.

Balanced Body's Pilates Program Video Series

- *BalancedBody's Pilates Mat Program*
- *Preparation for Balanced Body's Pilates Mat Program*
- *Polestar Beginning Mat Workout*
- *Polestar Intermediate Mat Workout*
- *Powerhouse Pilates Mat Program*

Physicalmind Institute®

- *Bodywork Matwork*
- *Cadillac Choreography*
- *Reform It!!!*

PowerHouse Pilates

- *Pilates Mat Program* with Marci Clark and Christine Romani-Ruby

STOTT PILATES™

- *22-minute Matwork*
- *Essential Matwork*
- *Intermediate Matwork*
- *Advanced Matwork*
- *Power Matwork*
- *Ultimate Back Care*
- *Flex-Band™ Workout*
- *Fitness Circle® Workout*
- *Power Fitness Circle®*

References

Behnke, Robert S. 2001. *Kinetic anatomy.* Champaign, IL: Human Kinetics.

Carrico, Mara. 1996. Five Fit Ways to Blend Body and Mind. *IDEA Today.* 14(April): 42–49.

Gallagher, Sean P., and Romana Kryzanowska, eds. 2000. *Joseph H. Pilates Archive Collection: The Photographs, Writings and Designs.* Philadelphia: Trans-Atlantic Publications.

Griffin, John C. 1998. *Client-centered exercise prescription.* Champaign, IL: Human Kinetics.

McGill, Stuart M. 2002. *Low back disorders: evidence-based prevention and rehabilitation.* Champaign, IL: Human Kinetics.

Norris, Christopher M. 2000. *Back stability.* Champaign, IL: Human Kinetics.

Pilates, Joseph H., and William J. Miller. [1945] 1998. *Pilates' Return to Life Through Contrology.* Edited by Judd Robbins. Incline Village, Nev.: Presentation Dynamics Inc.

SGMA International. 2002. *Tracking the Fitness Movement: 2002 Edition.* North Palm Beach, FL: Author.

U.S. Bureau of the Census. 2000. (NP-D1-A) *Projections of the Resident Population by Age, Sex, Race, and Hispanic Origin: 1999 to 2100.* Washington, D.C.

Watkins, James. 1999. *Structure and function of the musculoskeletal system.* Champaign, IL: Human Kinetics.

Additional Resources for Your Fitness Program

See the YMCA Program Store catalog for details about these additional items for your YMCA fitness program, or contact the Program Store, P.O. Box 5076, Champaign, IL 61825-5076, phone 800-747-0089. To save time, order by fax, 217-351-1549.
Please call if you are interested in receiving a free catalog.

Fitness Program Resources

0-88011-949-7	YMCA Personal Fitness Program Manual	$32.00
0-7360-3316-5	YMCA Fitness Testing and Assessment Manual (Fourth Edition)	$35.00
1-58518-029-7	Conducting the YMCA Fitness Testing and Assessment Protocol Video	$29.95
1-887781-00-5	Get Real: A Personal Guide to Real-Life Weight Management	$15.95
0-7360-0146-8	YMCA/IDEA Get Real Weight Management Program Instructor Manual	$19.00
0-88011-792-3	YMCA Fun and Fitness Activity Chart	$6.00
0-7360-1011-4	YMCA Heart Rate Check Poster	$17.00
1-58518-927-8	Exercise for Older Adults (ACE) (2E)	$37.95
0-99-003272-8	Xerball Instructor Manual	$20.00
0-99-003015-6	YogaBall Instructor Manual	$20.00
0-99-003123-3	Cycle Reebok: Professional Training Manual	$25.00
0-99-003013-X	Rubber Resistance Training Kit (Upper Body)	$30.00
0-99-003014-8	Rubber Resistance Training Kit (Lower Body)	$40.00
0-87322-717-4	YMCA Healthy Back Program Instructor's Guide	$23.00
0-87322-629-1	YMCA Healthy Back Book	$16.95
0-87322-692-5	YMCA Healthy Back Video	$24.95
0-88011-967-5	Exercises for a Healthy Back Poster	$17.00
0-88011-543-2	YMCA Walk Reebok Instructor Manual	$50.00
0-88011-899-7	YMCA Walk Reebok Distance/Interval Training Instructor Manual	$16.00

For a complete listing of all the fitness program resources, please refer to the Program Store catalog.

Prices shown are subject to change.